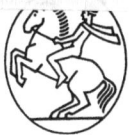

# Corneal Sensitivity

## Measurement and Clinical Importance

J. Draeger

with the collaboration of

M. Ackermann

H. Buhr-Unger

K. Hanke

K. Karjalainen

C. C. Kok-van-Alphen

H. Langenbucher

M. Lüders

R. Martin

B. Riss

E. Rumberger

W. Schloot

H. J. Völker-Dieben

R. Winter

Translated from the German
by F. C. Blodi

Springer-Verlag   Wien New York

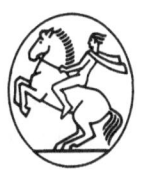

Prof. Dr. Jörg Draeger

Universitäts-Augenklinik Hamburg, Federal Republic of Germany

With 102 Figures

Library of Congress Cataloging in Publication Data. Draeger, Jörg. Corneal sensitivity. Includes bibliographical references and index. 1. Cornea – Diseases – Diagnosis. 2. Cornea – Sensitivity. 3. Cornea – Sensitivity – Measurement. I. Title. [DNLM: 1. Cornea – physiology. 2. Cornea – pathology. 3. Sensation – physiology. 4. Ophthalmology – instrumentation. WW 220 D758c.] RE336.D73. 1984. 617.7'19. 84-10602

ISBN-13:978-3-7091-8747-0      e-ISBN-13:978-3-7091-8745-6
DOI: 10.1007/978-3-7091-8745-6

# Foreword

We in ophthalmology are fortunate to be able to measure quantitatively many aspects of ocular morphology and visual function. These measurements are either objective (e. g. electroretinography, tonometry, electromyography, visually evoked responses, etc.) or subjective and psychophysical (e. g. visual acuity, visual fields, color vision, etc.).

One aspect of corneal physiology and pathology which has so far escaped careful and reliable measurements is corneal sensitivity. Previous attempts have been rather crude and can be compared to measuring intraocular pressure by digital compression.

Professor Draeger has for the last decade and a half directed his attention to the question of esthesiometry of the cornea. He has a gift for constructing and devising new ingenious ocular instruments. His handheld tonometer is a splendid example. He has now applied the principle of this instrument to the new electronic optical esthesiometer. In many publications he has reported on his first results using this modern technique to study corneal physiology and evaluate certain pathologic conditions.

In this monograph Professor Draeger has collected all of his material and reports on his long experience. The usefulness of this instrument is just beginning to be appreciated. It is obvious that this new measuring device will help us in the fitting of contact lenses, evaluating herpes simplex infections of the cornea, follow the postoperative course of patients with a penetrating keratoplasty, etc.

This is, obviously, only the first step in our evaluation of corneal sensitivity. An important beginning has been made and we are all indebted to Professor Draeger for initiating a new quantitative method which adds a new dimension to our ocular examinations. This method will prove to be valuable not only in ophthalmology, but also for neurology, neurosurgery and internal medicine.

Iowa City, Iowa, Winter 1984     Frederick C. Blodi, M. D.

# Contents

# 1. Introduction

The corneal sensitivity elicits one of the most sensitive defense reflexes of the human body. The threshold is unusually low, especially for the corneal center. This allows us to appreciate pathologic changes of this area early and with a high diagnostic reliability.

Basically, this has been known since the examination by Frey nearly 100 years ago. Difficulties in the methodology has so far prevented the esthesiometer to become useful in the clinic or in the daily practice. The thresholds are low and the stimuli have to be extremely delicate; the measurements must be quick and reproducible. These methodologic prerequisites have only recently been fulfilled.

A new wide field of experimental and clinical examinations has been opened with the new instrument. The results will be important, also outside the area of ophthalmology.

A renewed interest in the esthesiometry of the cornea was kindled by the increased frequency of viral infections. These have typically an influence on the corneal sensitivity. In addition, the esthesiometry may be of importance in the differential diagnosis of neurologic diseases.

Changes in corneal sensitivity may be of significance in glaucomatous eyes when they are being treated with beta blockers. The new method allows us to test exactly the effect of various surface anesthetics in regard to their concentration or composition.

The varying tolerance for contact lenses depends to some extent on the corneal sensitivity. On the other hand, the threshold for this sensitivity may be altered in patients who have worn contact lenses for a long period of time.

It has been known for quite some time that corneal sensitivity decreases after surgical interventions on the anterior segment of the eye. The sensitivity becomes normal with reinnervation of the surgical scar. Up to now this phenomenon could not be evaluated quantitatively. This phenomenon is important for the cataract operation, but especially significant for keratoplasties. The extent and the rate of reinnervation may differ whether a fresh cornea or a stored tissue is used.

Clinical experience has shown that after an extensive operation for a retinal detachment the anterior segment may undergo ischemic damages. We now can follow the extent and course of these pathologic changes by measuring the corneal sensitivity.

Changes in sensitivity will also occur with variations of the intraocular pressure. The extent and course of these changes could so far not be followed quantitatively.

The systemic metabolism will influence corneal sensitivity. This holds especially for diabetes mellitus. The effect of light coagulation treatment of a diabetic retinopathy may show unexpected alterations of corneal sensitivity.

This new instrument may enable us to measure metabolic influences during pregnancy.

There are also certain cases of genetic deviations from the normal corneal sensitivity.

This short list of clinical and experimental topics does not exhaust all possible application of esthesiometry. We are just at the beginning of our experiences with a new exact examination method which will yield not only scientific information, but will also be of diagnostic relevance for the clinic and the daily practice.

# 2. Anatomy and Physiology of the Cornea

## 2.1 Anatomy

### 2.1.1 The Layers of the Cornea

The human cornea is arranged in layers. These differ not only in their histologic morphologic aspect, but also from a physical chemical point of view.

The anterior border layer consists of several layers of non-keratinized squamous epithelium. Its basal membrane rests on Bowman's zone. The life cycle of an epithelial cell varies between six and seven days (Rohen, 1964). The tear film is attached to the epithelial surface by microvilli. The intercellular spaces are narrow and are closed

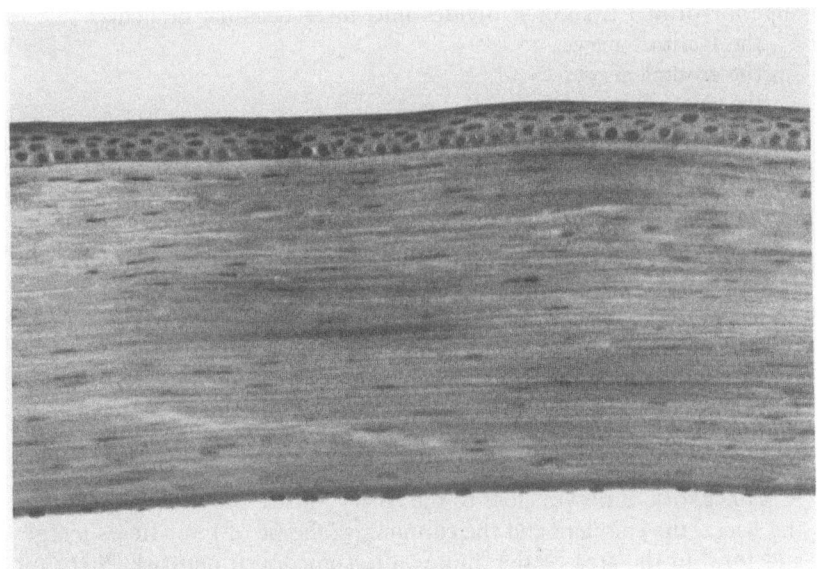

Fig. 1. The layers of the human cornea

by cytoplasmic cell bridges and desmosomes. There are numerous lipid deposits in the superficial epithelial layer. These deposits are derived from the meibomian glands (Ehlers, 1965). Bowman's zone represents an acellular homogeneous layer. Its anterior border is sharp, but posteriorly it merges with the rest of the stroma. Bowman's membrane is quite resistant to mechanical injuries. If damaged, it will regenerate only by the formation of scar tissue.

Seventy-five percent of the corneal stroma is water. It also contains a mucopolysaccharide ground substance; the concentration of $Na^+$ (172 mval) and $K^+$ (21 mval) differs from that in the epithelium. The collagen and elastic fibrils form numerous lamellae which are arranged parallel to the corneal surface. This arrangement of fibrils is much more regular in the cornea than in the sclera or in any other collagenous connective tissue. Among the lamellae are a few keratocytes. Descemet's membrane forms the posterior border toward the anterior chamber. It consists of a homogeneous layer of amorphous lamellae which are formed by the endothelial cells (Fig. 1).

## 2.1.2 Innervation of the Cornea

The first trigeminal branch provides the sensory innervation of the eyeball. The ophthalmic nerve originates in the Gasserian ganglion and then runs in the wall of the cavernous sinus. Before the nerve enters the superior orbital fissure, it divides into three terminal branches:

the lacrimal nerve,
the frontal nerve,
the nasociliary nerve.

The branches of the nasociliary nerves reach the globe, the mucous membrane of the posterior ethmoidal cells, the nose, the upper lid, the nasal canthus and the lacrimal sac. Two branches of this nerve innervate the eyeball (Waldeyer, 1975):

The Ramus communicans to the ciliary ganglion (the long root) carries sensory fibers to the globe.

There are approximately six short ciliary nerves which originate from the ganglion.

The long ciliary nerves course directly to the posterior pole of the eye.

These nerves penetrate the sclera close to the scleral canal of the optic nerve. They then run in the epichoroidal space forward (Fig. 2).

A network of nerves close to the ciliary muscle provides branches to the sclera, the episclera and the conjunctiva. Some of these fibers merge and form in the area of the limbus a circumcorneal network. Sixty to eighty myelinated nerves emanate from this network radially into the

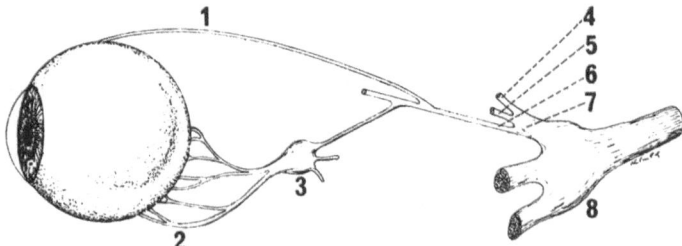

Fig. 2. Sensory innervation of the eyeball: *1* long ciliary nerves, *2* short ciliary nerves, *3* ciliary ganglion, *4* lacrimal nerve, *5* frontal nerve, *6* nasociliary nerve, *7* ophthalmic nerve, *8* gasserian ganglion

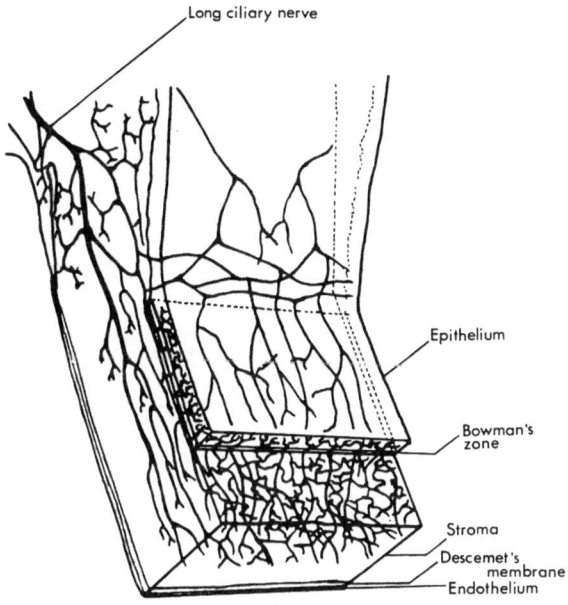

Fig. 3. Innervation of the cornea (after Hogan)

cornea. With few exceptions, the nerves lose their myelin sheaths as soon as they enter the corneal tissue (Zander and Weddell, 1951; Moses and Cotlier, 1970; Hogan, 1971).

These nerves preserve their schwannian elements up to their terminal branchings (Fig. 3).

Those parts of the nerves which are free of the schwannian sheath or where the schwannian sheath has gaps represent the receptor elements. The nerves penetrate into the stroma in various layers and form an anterior and a posterior network. Fine branches of the subepithelial net penetrate through pores of Bowman's membrane. The axons lose the schwannian sheath when entering the epithelial layer. At the same time the branches devide and some reach the superficial epithelial layer. We can therefore differentiate a basal network, ascending branches in the epithelium and superficial dendritic cells. On electron microscopic examination these terminal branches look like a string of pearls (Fig. 4).

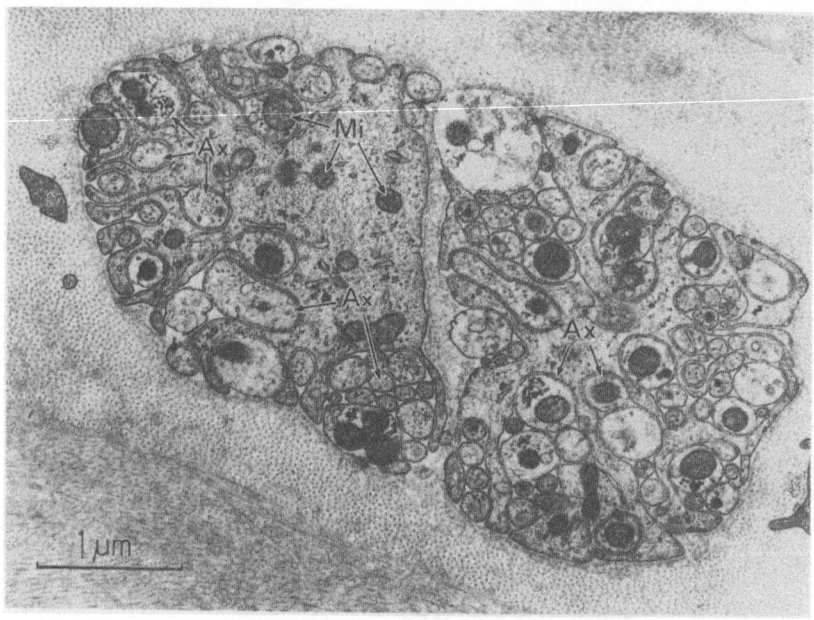

Fig. 4. Electron microscopic appearance of the corneal nerves (× 11,000)

The nerves of the corneal stroma come from the posterior network. The nerve endings lie mainly in the anterior stroma. They appear like small spherules, whereas the nerves themselves do not show any thickenings as described for the intraepithelial nerves. There are no nerves in Descemet's membrane and the endothelium.

The various morphologic appearance of the nerves has so far not been correlated with any functional differentiations, the exception being some thermal receptors at the limbus (Moses and Cotlier, 1970).

## 2.2. Corneal Sensitivity

There are specific receptors in the skin which transmit the various sensory modalities: The touch sensation is perceived via the corpuscles of Meissner and a network of nerves in the hair follicles; pressure is transmitted via the corpuscles of Vater-Pacini; the sensation of heat is perceived via the end organs of Ruffini and the sensation of cold by the end bulbs of Krause. Only pain is transmitted via free nerve endings in the epidermis. These specific receptors are not found in the cornea. We only find free nerve endings which come from fine terminal branches of mixed or long ciliary nerves. They terminate with a bulb-like thickening in the anterior stroma or in the epithelium In spite of the lack of any specific receptors the corneal nerve endings may transmit pain, touch, cold and heat sensations.

The density of the innervational network is highest in the center of the cornea encompassing an area of 5 mm in diameter. The density decreases toward the limbus. There are more free nerve endings in the horizontal meridian than in the vertical one, and more in the temporal half than in the nasal one.

In the past touch could not be differentiated from pain and only a single threshold could be established (Strughold, 1930). In more recent investigations with delicate stimuli, touch and pain can be differentiated (Lele and Weddell, 1956). However, different receptors are not found; both sensations are transmitted via free nerve endings (Mark and Maurice, 1977).

The nerve fibers can be differentiated into slow conducting, not adapting C-fibers and into fast conducting A-delta-fibers which transmit a high frequency pulse (Burgess and Perl, 1973) which on repeated stimulation become inactive (Perl, 1971).

There is no sensation for heat or cold in the cornea. These sensations are confined to the conjunctiva (Bevermann *et al.*, 1973) or originate by heat conduction to the thermoreceptors of the iris (Dawson, 1963).

# 3. Development of the Various Methods of Esthesiometry

## 3.1 Early Investigations

M. von Frey presented in 1894 in his publication "Contribution to the physiology of pain" the first "esthesiometer." "A hair or a piece of it which should be as little curved as possible, is attached to the end of a light wood rod of about 8 cm length. The hair lies vertical to the axis of the rod so that it will on one side protrude for 20–30 mm, under certain circumstances even more. Such a rod presents with appropriate application a stimulus of definite and permanent value. If the hair is now placed vertically on the skin surface, a pressure will be exerted which cannot exceed a certain limit." (Fig. 5.)

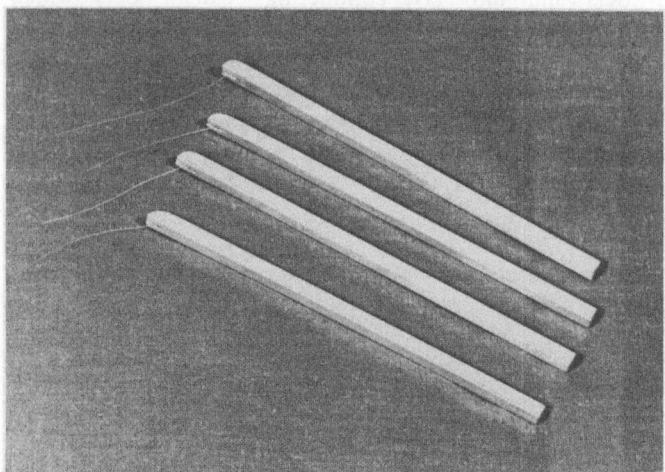

Fig. 5. v. Frey's hair

v. Frey examined with this instrument his own eyes while observing the procedure in a mirror. Unfortunately, it has been shown that some important part of v. Frey's postulates are not fulfilled:

These hairs do not present a "stimulus of definite and permanent value." The rigidity of such a hair, which is the measured value, depends not only on the condition and age of the hair, but especially upon air humidity, and room temperature at the time of the measurement. An important factor is also the speed with which the hair is approached to the surface, as well as the angle under which it meets the surface.

Further quantitative examinations which were also done by v. Frey showed that there is a certain individual range of responses; there are also considerable topographic differences of the corneal threshold values for various stimuli: "The threshold of the cornea lies around 0.3 gm/mm². In most areas the touch with a hair is not felt at all, whereas at some points a slight sensation may be perceived. These sensitive points are evenly distributed over the corneal surface and can be found in the center as well as near the limbus."

We now know that these conclusions by v. Frey are based on inadequacies of his method. A truly quantitative reproducible topographic measurement was at that time not possible.

Marx (1925) performed further examinations with v. Frey's hair. When examining the distribution of sensitive points, he found that in general the temporal half of the cornea is more sensitive than the nasal half, the lower half more than the upper one and the center is about 60% more sensitive than the periphery.

Goldscheider and Brückner (1919) also published results which deviated from the ones obtained by v. Frey. They used not only hair, but also cotton wisps and metal probes in order to differentiate the pain of touch and the sensation of heat. They also initiated experiments on the effect of surface anesthetics.

Marinosci (1930) obtained threshold values similar to those of v. Frey. He used 5 cm long horsehair of varying lengths. Morinaga (1931) determined in the corneal center a threshold of 0.1 gm/mm², in the periphery 1.5 gm/mm². His sensitivity threshold was therefore much lower than that found by v. Frey.

## 3.2 Newer Attempts for a Technical Solution

Cerise (1908) was the first to obtain a direct measure of the individual strength of the stimulus: "The stimulus is exerted by an exchangeable hair. The resistance which is exerted by the hair when placing it and when it bends is increased by a connected spiral spring. This resistance can be measured on a dial and then checked on a scale and expressed in mm." He performed with this instrument measurements on various corneal diseases, but also after cataract extractions. He noted the decreased sensitivity for touch central from the area of the surgical incision, while the rest of the cornea had a normal sensitivity threshold. Cerise also tested the influence of various drugs on the touch sensitivity of the cornea.

In spite of the attempts to measure with a spring force this instrument had the same principal disadvantages as v. Frey's method –

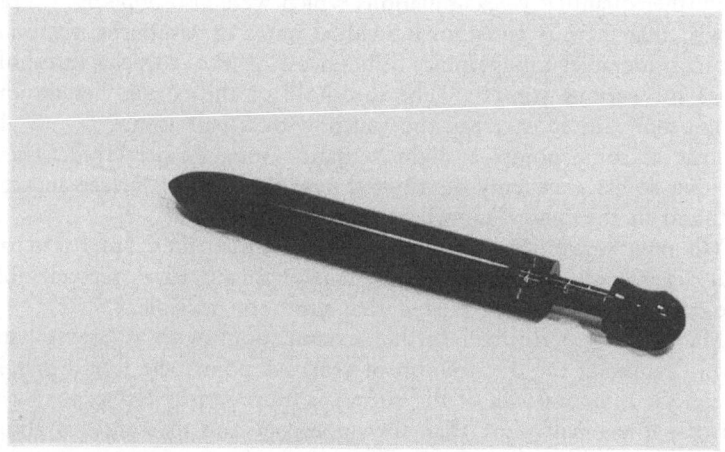

Fig. 6. The esthesiometer with a nylon thread of Boberg-Ans

the humidity of the air and the room temperature strongly influenced the rigidity of the hair.

Boberg-Ans published in 1956 his modification of the v. Frey method: A nylon thread in a copper handle was used. The free end of this thread was exchangeable (Fig. 6).

This method allows us to change the rigidity of the stimulus in a definite way. Boberg-Ans examined the threshold values in young and old patients, after perforating injury, after caustic burns, and in the area of corneal ulcers. He emphasized the loss of corneal sensitivity in herpetic keratitis, examined the condition in hereditary corneal dystrophies and in keratitis and scleritis.

Boberg-Ans was the first to use the esthesiometer for the fitting of contact lenses.

In some other studies he explored the possibility of measuring corneal sensitivity with an airstream. He finally had to abandon this attempt because air turbulence interefered with the results.

Sugita (1977) and Rasch (1982) experimented with an "airstream esthesiometer." They did not report on any clinical experiences.

Lele and Weddell (1956) also attempted to use an airstream as a stimulus. They used varying temperatures by selecting infrared rays of one or three microns. These can be directed at definite corneal areas.

Another improvement of the Boberg-Ans instrument is being produced since 1961 in France following a suggestion by Cochet and Bonnet (Fig. 7).

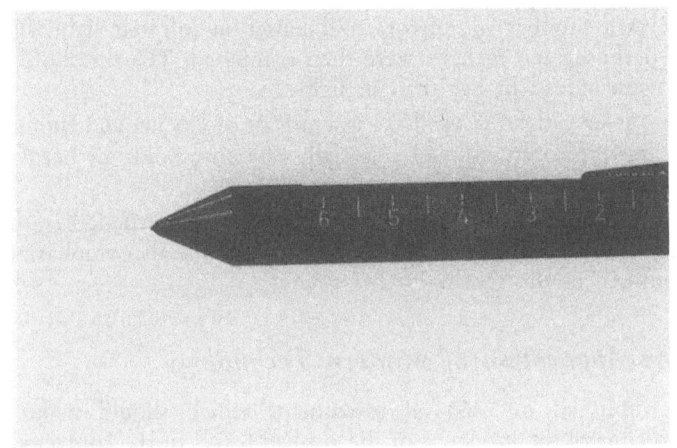

Fig. 7. Esthesiometer with a thread according to Cochet and Bonnet

The threshold values found with this instrument lie on an average at 10 mg in the corneal center and at 18 mg in the periphery. In general, they confirm the results obtained by Boberg-Ans and by v. Frey. Cochet and Bonnet complement these results by some practical hints:

1. The coefficient of elasticity can be altered by the air humidity and by dipping the thread too long into a disinfectant solution.
2. Drying of the cornea will increase the threshold of corneal sensitivity.
3. If the corneal sensitivity is low and if the nylon thread is short and therefore rigid, the procedure may produce a small epithelial defect which can be demonstrated by using fluorescein and the corneal microscope.
4. We have to differentiate the periodic involuntary lid blink from a lid blink which is a defense reflex, especially in apprehensive patients.
5. The examination should begin at the upper limbus in order to demonstrate to the patient that the procedure is painless.
6. The lashes should not be touched during the procedure.

Couchet and Bonnet (1960) reported about their results in various corneal affections, also in trachoma. They studied changes of corneal sensitivity after wearing contact lenses.

Bonnet and Millodot (1965) examined how the optical impression of the approaching hair can influence the measurements. Ten patients were measured in complete darkness. The instrument was mounted on a slit lamp. The site of application and the bending of the thread were observed via a number of mirrors and lenses in infrared light. The results in darkness and in light were then compared. The threshold in darkness were indeed higher than in light.

Numerous investigators used the instrument of Cochet and Bonnet, e. g. Severin, 1965. She studied especially the thresholds in herpetic keratitis.

Norn (1970) also used this instrument to examine herpetic keratitis and found a characteristic decrease of sensitivity. He also emphasized that age influences the sensitivity for touch.

## 3.2.1 The Application of Modern Technology

Schirmer published in 1963 an instrument which should make it possible to control the influence of the applied force, of the contact site and friction. The applied force could be read on a small scale (Fig. 8).

The contact surface can be varied by using small plastic discs of different diameter. The measurements are performed while the patient is in a supine position. First the touch and then the pain threshold are determined. In order to determine the friction of the stimulus on the corneal surface the patient had to change his direction of gaze during the measurement. With the same force a lower threshold will be obtained if the contact surface becomes larger. Schirmer devised a "pressure index" in order to define the total applied stimulus. He explained his results as a summation of impulses in the tested area.

Larson (1970) devised the first electromagnetic esthesiometer. He aimed to avoid the above mentioned disadvantages of using a thread. The instrument was constructed by Larson and Millodot and had a measuring point consisting of a double bent fine platinum wire of an exactly determined diameter.

The point of the wire approaches the cornea automatically with constant speed. The exerted force can be varied continuously between 1–200 mg. The platinum point is attached to a torsion wire and is moved with an electrical motor. When the corneal surface is touched, a photocell disengages the motor and the platinum wire is withdrawn by spring action into its original position.

The authors compare their results with those of Cochet and Bonnet. Clinical results were not published. Razichovskij (1971) described a magnetic "algesimeter." The force necessary to determine the threshold value in measured with the help of magnetic friction of a stimulus which slides within a sheath.

Regina Gotz (1972) constructed two new measuring instruments. She called one an „electromillidynamometer." The other one was a spring esthesiometer, similar to the one devised by Schirmer in 1963. It was equipped with exchangeable springs of varying strength so that a measuring scale between 0 to 10 mg, 10 to 20 mg or 20 to 30 mg could be chosen.

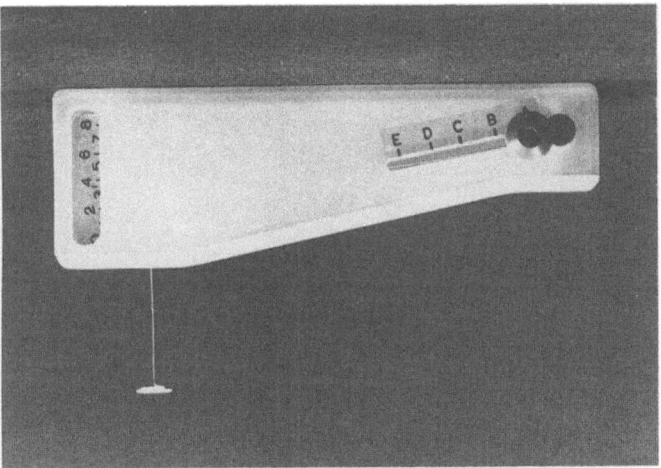

Fig. 8. Esthesiometer of Schirmer

The "electromillidynamometer" is equipped with two measuring devices, one for the range of 10 to 100 mg and the other one for a range of 100 to 500 mg. The exerted force is measured on a millivolt meter. The threshold values obtained with this instrument lie between 10.5 and 11.1 mg, though there are no statements about the size of the measuring device or the topographic differences. Clinical results were not reported. A mechanical esthesiometer was constructed in 1967 (Draeger). It is based on the principle of the mechanical optical applanation tonometer. It was supposed to give more reproducible results. The measuring force – similar to a handheld applanation tonometer – was here produced by a spiral spring the tension of which could continuously be controlled by an electrical motor. Illumination and observation were similar to those of a handheld applanation tonometer. The range corresponded to the values which were to be expected in esthesiometry: At first a range of 0 to 2 p was suggested. When this device was tested it could be shown that the desired force could be obtained with a high precision. On the other hand, the test body had in comparison to the force a considerable mass which led to a disturbing resonance. This made the measurements practically difficult. It was not possible to dampen these autoresonance vibrations of the highly sensitive system by purely mechanical means (Fig. 9).

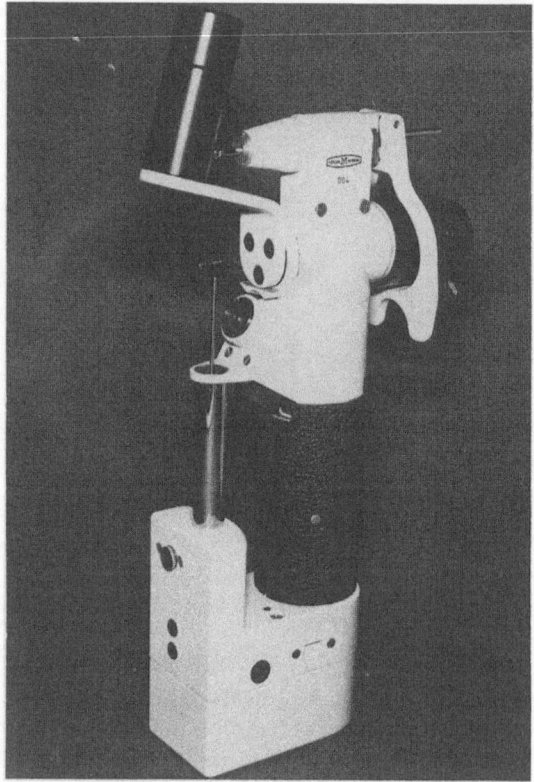

Fig. 9. Electromechanical hand esthesiometer (Draeger, 1967)

## 3.3 Electronic-Optic Esthesiometer

The numerous previous attempts to solve the problem of a quantitative reproducible esthesiometry had been futile; it had not been possible to develop a clinically useful, precise and simple instrument.

We tried on the basis of our previous experiences with the mechanical optical esthesiometer a new device using modern electronic technology. The following requirements should be met:

1. High precision of the measurements, independent of the air humidity or room temperature, independent of the skill of the examiner.
2. Optical control of the contact between the measuring device and the corneal surface in order to determine definitely the site of impact.
3. A continuous range of force between 0 and $500 \times 10^{-5}$ N (with the possibility to extent the range upward); the error range, especially for the lower forces, should be as small as possible.
4. The possibility to perform the esthesiometry with a predetermined stimulus strength, corresponding to the previous experiences obtained with the instrument of v. Frey.
5. The possibility of a "dynamic esthesiometry" with a continuous increase of force while the instrument remains in contact with the cornea.
6. Automatic advancement at a predetermined speed of the stimulus toward the corneal surface; a ballistic effect during the time of impact has to be avoided.
7. One should be able to use the device quickly and simply; the measurement should be obtained within the interval of a physiologic blink.
8. The stimulus should have a definite size and surface contour; it should have minimal heat conduction.
9. It should be easy to sterilize the test body.
10. There should be absolutely no danger of injuring the patient.

A prototype was built that could be used with the slit lamp table; this made it possible to move the test body on the joystick device with the help of a motor which could control the head rest. This made precise positioning possible (Fig. 10).

It was important to determine the point of contact precisely. This would make it possible to plot a topographic threshold profile of the cornea. Especially useful was the motor driven chin rest device which was synchronized with adjustments of the stool. The test body was viewed obliqued from the side. The force was regulated with two push buttons. The resulting force was presented digitally with two light diodes enabling the examiner to read instantaneously the force exerted by the test body at a definite time.

Another button initiated the movement of the test body. The device approaches the corneal surface automatically with a predetermined speed. The examiner, therefore, does not have to touch the instrument during this maneuver at all. When contact with the cornea has been established, the predetermined force is exerted. When calculating the surface of the test body, we recognized that this surface should at a minimum be larger than the distance between two free nerve endings, which is at least 10 microns. A number of physical problems arises when a stimulus of such small surface is being used:

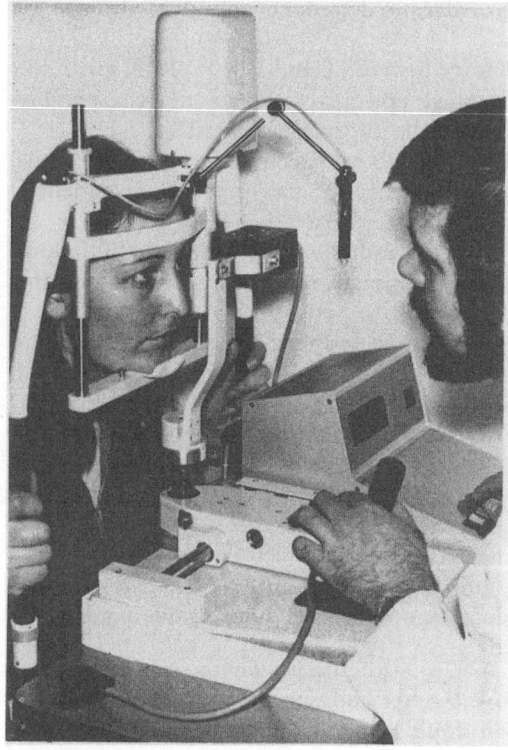

Fig. 10. Electronic esthesiometer mounted on a slit lamp table

Pressure equals force per surface unit; if the surface is extremely small even a minimal force will produce relatively high pressures. This means that the mechanical requirements for the measuring device would be especially high as unusually small forces have to be used. Such stimuli with small surface represent an increased risk of injuring the corneal epithelium.

On the other hand, too large a surface of the stimulus could also lead to inaccurate results. Because of the convex surface of the cornea, the contact area could not be unequivocally defined. In addition, the pressure extended within this area would vary. Too large a stimulus surface would not allow an accurate topographic esthesiometry.

We therefore decided to test in some pilot studies the optimal surface size of the test body and varied the diameter from 1.0 to 0.5 to 0.3 to 0.1 mm. The test body was blackened with a matt lacquer in order to avoid an optical irritation of the patient by the approaching stimulus.

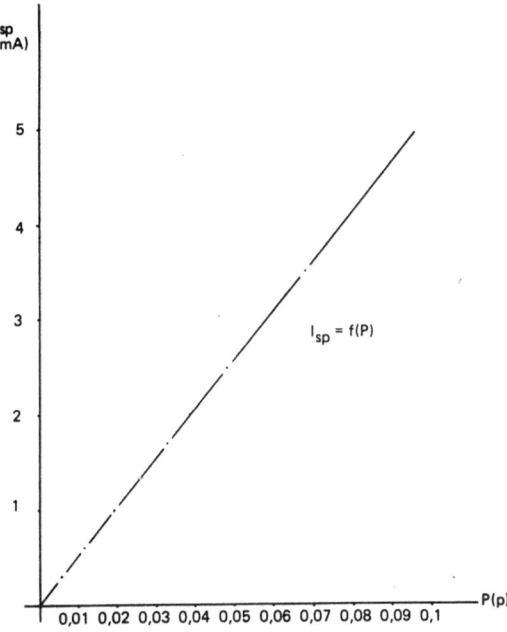

Fig. 11. Calibration curve 0–0.1 p

The instrument was calibrated by measuring the produced force as indicated by the current on a highly sensitive analytical balance. We achieved a practically linear correlation over the entire range of measurements up to 1.0 p, and especially in the lower range of 0.00 to 0.1 p, which is for our measurements especially important.

In order to correspond to the new international nomenclature, the digital values were indicated in $1 \times 10^{-5} N$ ($1 N = 1.02 \times 10^{-1}$ kp) (Figs. 11 and 12).

The technical characteristics of the prototype proved to be sufficient to achieve our desired scientific goals, especially to obtain a

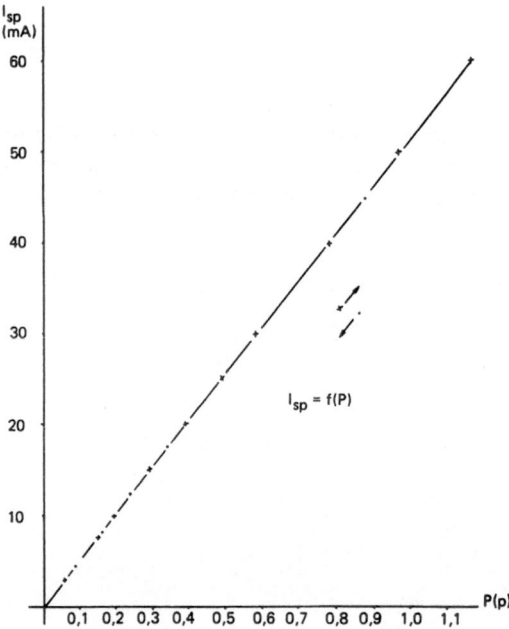

Fig. 12. Calibration curve 0.1–1.0 p

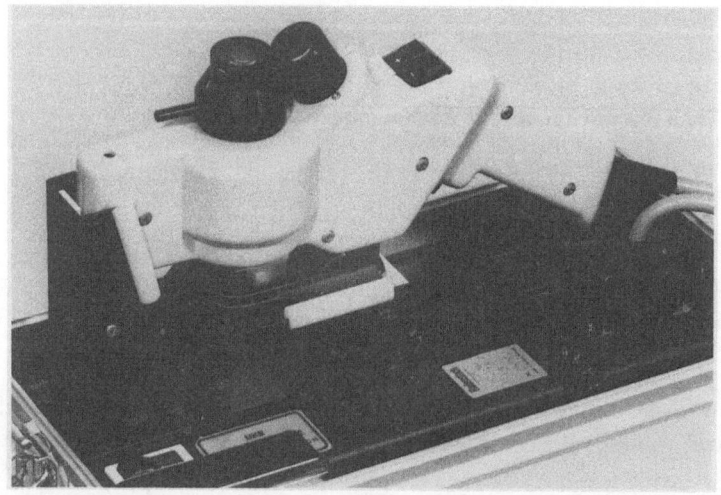

Fig. 13. Electronic optic handheld esthesiometer

topographic threshold profile and to examine age-dependent threshold values.

An instrument which was not easily movable seemed impractical for clinical use. This first prototype was not suitable for clinical practice nor for the study of special cases in the neurologic, neurosurgical or internal clinic.

We have therefore developed an instrument which is movable and handheld. This new instrument was modeled along the experiences obtained with the previously designed handheld applanation tonometer (Fig. 13).

## 3.3.1 Producing and Measuring the Stimulus Force

The instrument consists of a part held by the examiner's hand and a part resting on a table; the latter part contains an electric governing device and a sterilization attachment. Both parts are connected by an electric wire (Fig. 14).

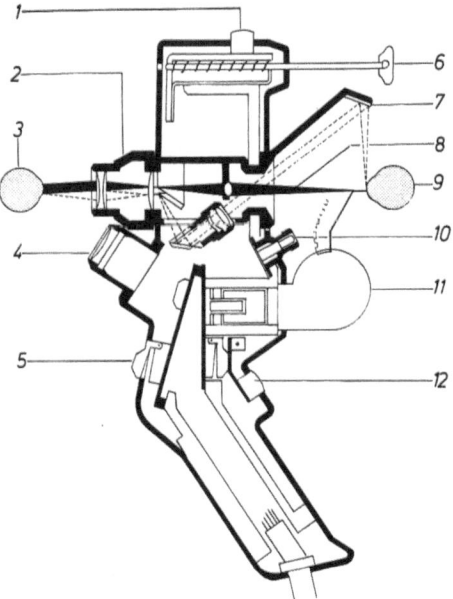

Fig. 14. Schematic cross-section through the electronic optic esthesiometer. *1* Release button for frontal suggest, *2* Observation ocular, *3* Examiner's eye, *4* Force control, *5* Buttons to change the amount of force exerted, *6* Frontal support, *7* Lateral observation, *8* Vertical observation, *9* Patient's eye, *10* Illumination, *11* Measuring device with stimulus body, *12* Start button

The core of the measuring device is a small moving coil galvanometer as it is used to measure weak direct electric currents. Here it is used to produce a force which is via a lever, the stimulus body, exerted on the cornea (Fig. 15).

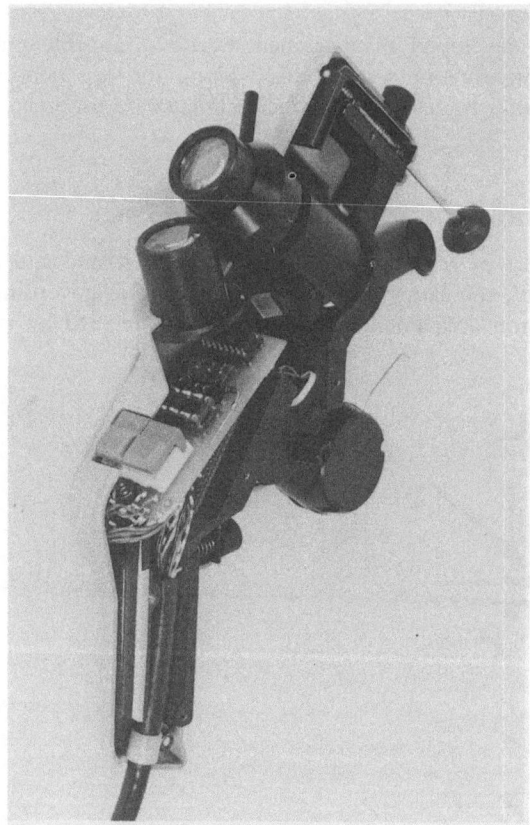

Fig. 15. Design of the electronic-optical esthesiometer

In order to explain the origin of this force of few principal properties of the moving coil galvanometer have to be recalled.

Such a galvanometer consists essentially of a rectangular copper wire coil which is attached to a suspension which can be rotated, plus a concentrically constructed permanent magnet. The coil is freely movable in a small air slit between the two poles of the magnet. Because of the concentric construction the magnetic field in the air slit is radially arranged. This magnetic field permeates vertically the part of the coil which lies between the two poles. When a direct electric current of an intensity i flows through the coil, a rotary force Ne will be exerted on the coil following the laws of electrodynamics (Lorentz). The coil will be rotated out of its position of rest. The following relation will apply for a rotatory force Ne, a current intensity i, a magnetic induction B and a coil surface A:

$$Ne = n \cdot A \cdot B \cdot i$$

The direction of rotation is determined by the direction of the magnetic field and of the electric current. By this rotation of the coil a counterrotation Nm of the suspension will be produced. This counterrotation is directly proportional to the deviation angle $\varrho$ from the position of rest of the coil:

$$Nm = -D \cdot \varrho$$

D is a constant of the suspension attachment.

At a definite angle of deviation $\varrho$, the counterrotation Nm is equal but opposite to the rotatory force Ne. Both forces cancel each other and the coil acquires at $\varrho$, a new position of rest:

$$Ne = Nm = 0$$

A, B, D and n are constant for a specific instrument and the deviation angle $\varrho$ depends therefore only on the intensity of the current; it is directly proportional to it. If we now attach an indicator to the coil, this arrangement can be used to measure a direct current.

The esthesiometer works on a similar principle. The force which presses the stimulus body against the cornea is produced in a moving coil instrument. Instead of an indicator (as used in a galvanometer), we have here the stimulus body firmly attached to the coil. The length of the lever of the stimulus body is constant and therefore the force exerted at the tip of the stimulus body is directly proportional to the rotatory movement of the coil.

As soon as the tip of the test body encounters the cornea it cannot advance anymore. The angle of deviation remains constant and the counterrotatory motion Nm cannot increase anymore. Any further increase of the current in the coil will result in a force which cannot be compensated anymore by the suspension device, but will be directly exerted on the cornea. This enables us to control the force exerted on the cornea by regulating the intensity of the current.

In order to avoid any force of gravity which could exert an additional undesired rotatory force on the revolving coil the entire rotatory system of the esthesiometer (coil, stimulus body and suspension) is balanced by counterweights. This enables us to use the instrument in any position, i.e. we are independent from the position of the patient at the time of the examination. The examination can be precisely performed on a sitting or on a lying patient.

The intensity of the current determines therefore the rotatory movement of the coil and thereby the force exerted by the stimulus body. By regulating the current we regulate the force exerted by the stimulus body on the cornea. The correct amount of the current has to flow through the coil to enable a measurement at a definite time. This is regulated by a microprocessor which is in the governing part of the instrument and which can be programmed for that purpose.

We distinguish four main positions for the dynamic method (Fig. 16):

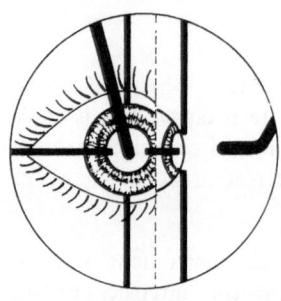

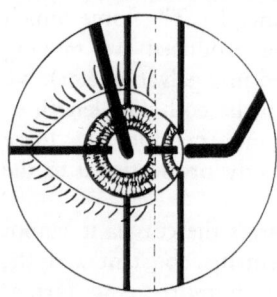

Fig. 16. Main positions of the contact pin of the electronic-optic esthesiometer observed through the aiming device

Position 1: The stimulus body is in contact with the instrument
Position 2: Contact pin while approaching
Position 3: Contact pin touching the corneal centre
Position 4: The stimulus body reverses to the end position (about 1 mm behind position 3).

The microprocessor is programmed in such a way that the following movements will result:

When the instrument is switched the stimulus body moves into position 1. By pressing the "start" button in the handle of the instrument the stimulus body moves quickly (in about 1 sec.) into position 2. From here the mechanism proceeds in slow motion (duration maximally 3 sec.) into position 3. This decreases to a minimum the dynamic force when the stimulus body encounters the cornea (Fig. 17).

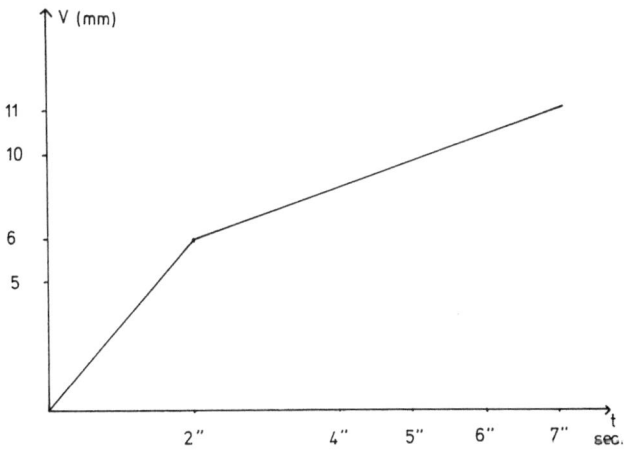

Fig. 17. Stepwise decrease in the speed of the test body approaching the cornea

By now using the "+" or the "−" buttons (which are also located in the handle) the force exerted on the cornea can be continuously increased or decreased. As long as one of these buttons is pressed down, the exerted force will keep on increasing or decreasing. The change of force is in the interval 0 to $100 \times 10^{-5}$N linear with time, in the interval 100 to $1000 \times 10^{-5}$N exponential with time. Both intervals take about three seconds. The exerted force can be read off a digital LED-indicator (Fig. 18).

When the start button is released the stimulus body returns to position 1. The last achieved force remains visible in the digital indicator until the "+" or "−" buttons are pressed again.

The patient's response has in this "subjective" measurement a certain latency which is a defect of the system; this defect will remain proportional to the force exerted. This arrangement will also decrease the duration of a measurement when the threshold is high so that the measurement can still be taken within the interval of a physiologic blink. This is especially important for the so-called "dynamic" esthesiometry in which the test device rests on the cornea during the entire phase of increasing force.

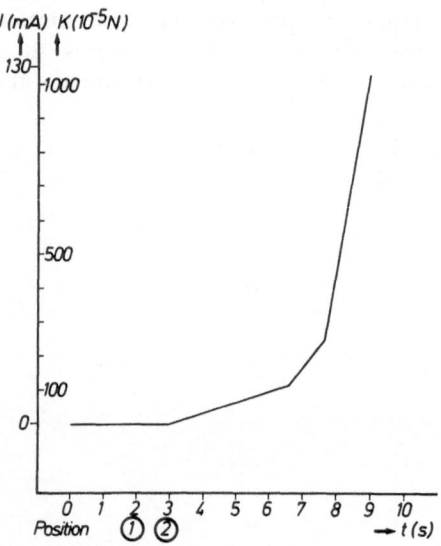

Fig. 18. Nonlinear increase of force during the measurement

For the so-called static method a certain force can be predetermined by pushing the "+" or "−" buttons before the esthesiometer advances toward the eye. When the start button is pushed the stimulus body again goes into positions 2 and 3. In contrast to the dynamic method the "+" and "−" buttons are here not used.

While the start button is still pressed down the preset force will be reached within a fraction of a second once position 3 has been gained and this preset force will now be exerted on the cornea. If one now wishes to increase or decrease this force the "+" or "−" buttons have to be pushed. The digital indicator will show the preset force, or the actual force if the "+" or "−" buttons have been used.

In some early instruments, which differed in some technical details from the later series, we actually registered the course of movements as the test body advances toward the cornea (Fig. 19).

The measurement comprises the interval from the position of rest to the maximal deviation and then back again until the lever has reached its original position. The time necessary for the entire measurement is

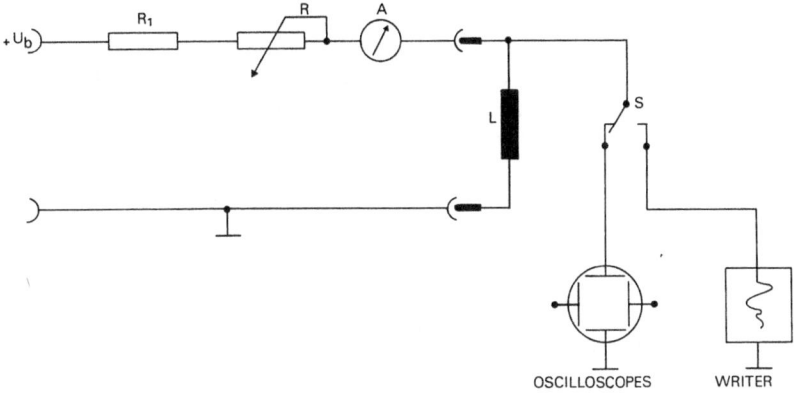

Fig. 19. Measuring device for the registration of the movement of the testing body

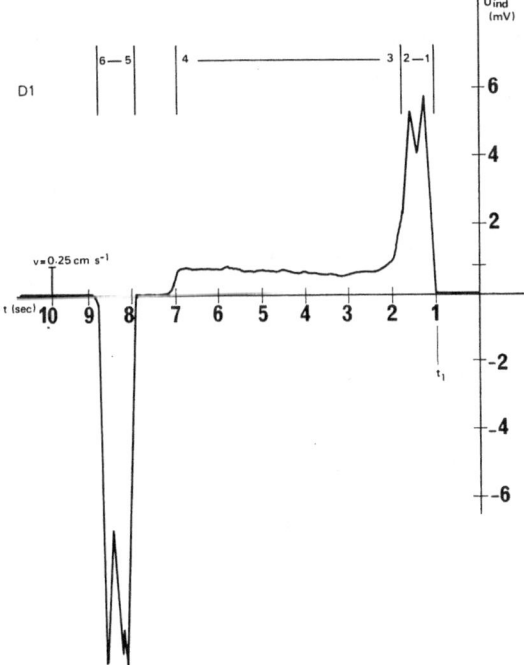

Fig. 20. Oscillographic representation of the speed with which the test body moves

six seconds when the speed with which the instrument moves toward the cornea lies between 0.8 and 1 cm per second$^{-1}$, or 0.2 and 0.25 cm per second$^{-1}$ (Fig. 20).

The first two spikes represent the beginning of the measurement, i.e. the disc begins to turn. The lever remains for a short time in its resting position because of the impedence of its mass. It follows the movement somewhat later. When the disc has reached a low speed of rotation, the lever is firmly positioned and decreases its speed of movement. The actual measurement begins after three seconds. The test object has now reached its average speed of 0.25 cm per second$^{-1}$. The contact with the cornea should occur with this speed. At four the maximal deviation of the test body has been reached, five and six signify its withdrawal to the original position. In order to evaluate the ballistic impact when the test body touches the cornea, we have to observe the dynamic behavior of the lever. Every mass possesses at a definite speed a certain kinetic energy. The lever of this instrument has a rotatory energy which depends upon the resistance of the mass and the angular speed of the lever. In the instant the test body touches the cornea, the lever is dampened so that its energy of motion will be transmitted to the area of contact. When the impulse of the force tapers off, this elastic deformation will be partially retransmitted to the lever system. This may produce a resonance.

It was now our aim to modify the course of motion in such a way that the test body remains after the impact in contact with the corneal epithelium without showing any reverbations. Several factors had to be considered in order to achieve this goal:
1. the strength of the impulse of the force (kinetic energy),
2. the strenth of the dampening force (predetermined amount of force in the instrument),
3. the friction of the lever,
4. the capillary adhesion between the test body and the precorneal tear film,
5. the corneal elasticity.

Factors 2 to 4 would dampen the resonance. The next objective was to estimate the impulse of the force. In the moment of impact the test body has the rotatory energy E. Energy means that work can be produced, in our case the work produced by the deformation ($W = F \times \triangle s$); it therefore follows:

$$E = \frac{1}{2} \times J \times \omega^2 = F \times \triangle s = W$$

$$F = \frac{1}{\triangle s} \times \frac{1}{2} J \times \omega^2$$

transformed toward F
W  = the work necessary for the deformation
$\triangle s$ = deviation of the center of gravity
F   = impacting force

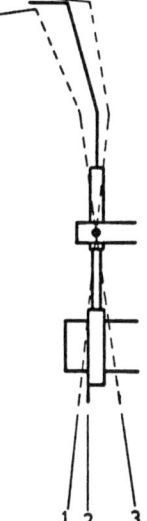

1 = Position at rest
2 = Position at contact with cornea
3 = Maximal deviation

Fig. 21. Dynamic of the lever system

In order to determine the unknown factor (J) the lever is suspended at a definite point (Λ) and then touched so that it starts to swing. The swinging duration T is measured and the mass of the entire lever system is determined (see Fig. 21). The impedence can be determined by the following formulas:

$$T = 2\pi \ \frac{m}{c} = 2 \ \frac{J_a}{G_e} \qquad\qquad J = J_2 - m \ e^2$$

$$J_a = G_e \left(\frac{T}{2\pi}\right)^2 \qquad\qquad G_e = m \ g \ e$$

$$J = G_e \left(\frac{T}{2\pi}\right)^2 - m \times e^2 = m \times g \ e \ \left(\frac{T}{2\pi}\right)^2 - m \ e^2$$

T  = duration of swinging = 0.57 seconds
$G_e$ = moment when lever returns
m  = mass = 2.56 gram
$J_a$ = the amount of impedence in A
e  = length = 76 mm

$$J = 2.56 \times 981 \times 7.6 \left(\frac{0.57}{2\pi}\right)^2 = 2.56 \times 7.6^2 \text{ g} \times s^2 \times s^{-2} \text{ cm} \times \text{cm}$$

$$\underline{J = 9.81 \text{ g cm}^2}$$

$$E = \frac{1}{2} J\omega^2 \qquad \omega = \frac{v}{e} \qquad\qquad v = \text{speed of impact} = 0.2 \text{ cm/sec.}$$

$$\omega = 0.026 \qquad e = \text{length} = 7.6 \text{ cm}$$

$$E = \frac{1}{2} 9.81 \times 0.026^2 \text{ g cm}^2 g^{-2}$$

$$\underline{E = 0.0033 \text{ g cm}^2 g^{-2}}$$

$$F = \frac{1}{\varDelta s} \times E = \frac{1}{50 \times 10} -4 \times 0.0033 = 0.66 \text{ g cm } s^{-2} = \underline{0.66 \times 10^{-5} \text{ N}}$$

.    The test body makes at first contact with the precorneal tear film. Already at that time a stimulus is transmitted to the cornea itself. Corresponding to the surface tension of the tear fluid a more or less potent adhesion force will be exerted between the test body and the fluid. If this adhesion force is stronger than the one exerted by the lacrimal fluid, the test body will be wetted and the fluid will be pulled upward along the test body. At this moment there is nearly a "negative" force between the test body and the corneal surface, i.e. a suction force. The strength of this capillary force can be measured on a sensitive analytical balance (Fig. 22).

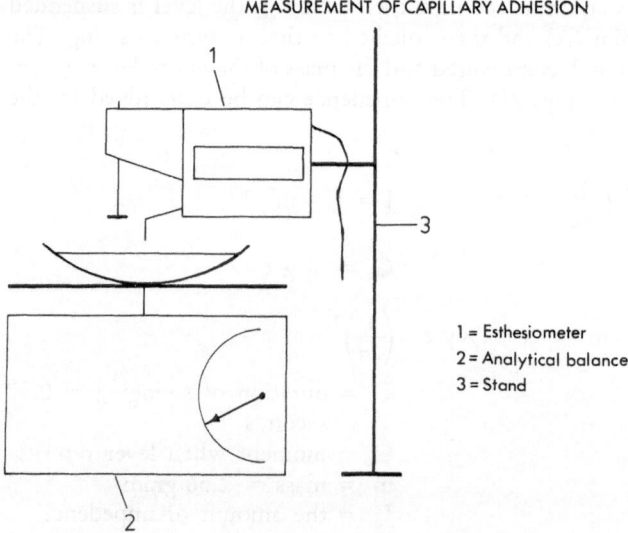

MEASUREMENT OF CAPILLARY ADHESION

1 = Esthesiometer
2 = Analytical balance
3 = Stand

Fig. 22. Experimental design to measure the capillary adhesion between the test body and the corneal surface

The mean value of 10 mesurements showed that this force is $0.25 \pm 0.05 \times 10^{-5}\,\mathrm{N}$.

## 3.3.2 The Optical Device for the Observation

A special optical device allows the observer to view simultaneously the area to be tested and the exact time at which the measurement is obtained. One objective and a mirror image the cornea laterally from the corneal vertex. The surface of the eye is imaged frontally by the objective L1 (Fig. 23) and the ocular L2. The objective L1 produces a minified real inverted image which lies in the focal plane of the ocular.

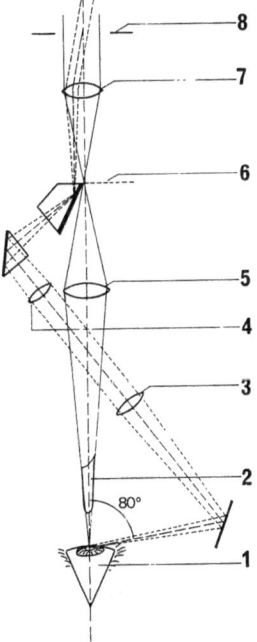

Fig. 23. Design of the observation optics: *1* the eye of the patient, *2* the body, *3* Objective for the lateral image f = 80, *4* Objective for the lateral image f = 40, *5* Objective for the main image f = 25, *6* Reticule, *7* Ocular f = 25, *8* Position of exit pupil

At this place a graduated plate is placed which presents auxiliary markings in order to guarantee an optimal range for the motion of the test body. An image of the corneal vertex profile is placed laterally into the path of the rays. This image is produced by a movable mirror (Fig. 24).

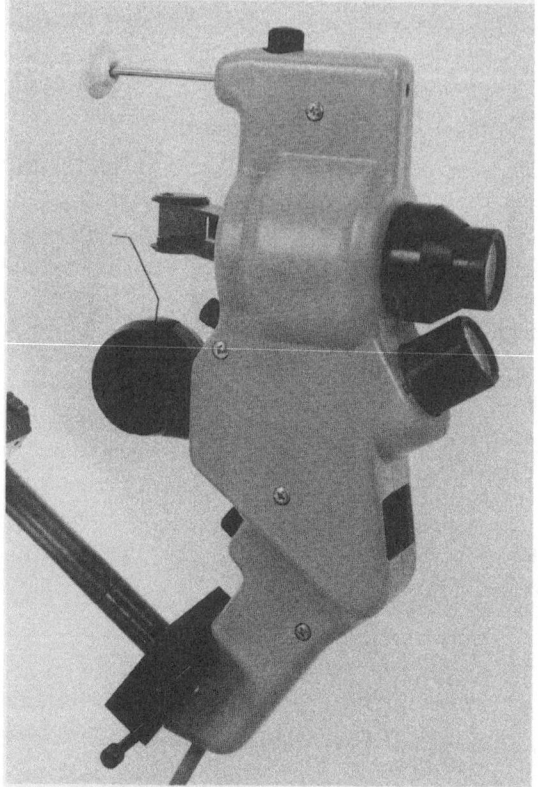

Fig. 24. Head of the esthesiometer with front rest, test body, mirror tubes and illumination

The distance between the ocular and the eye of the patient should be 34 mm corresponding to the location of the exit pupil. At this distance the main image and the laterally superimposed image of the corneal vertex can be viewed simultaneously. The ocular can be adjusted to the refractive error of the observer (Fig. 25).

This system allows to choose a specific area for the measurement, to control the exact time of the measurement, to recognize a possible tilting of the test body or any disturbing ocular movements.

The observation is facilitated by a built-in illumination system. A low voltage lamp illuminates the cornea at an angle of 30°. The condenser is a special bulb with a profile glass soldered on. This works like a condenser and delineates the illumination cone. The intensity of the illumination should be capable of resolving the microscopic picture without annoying the patient; nor should it increase his blink frequency which would make the measurements more difficult. The heat produced by the illumination system could during prolonged measurements lead to a superficial dessication of the cornea. This illumination system is dazzling enough so that the approaching test body with its matt lacquered surface will hardly be noticed by the patient.

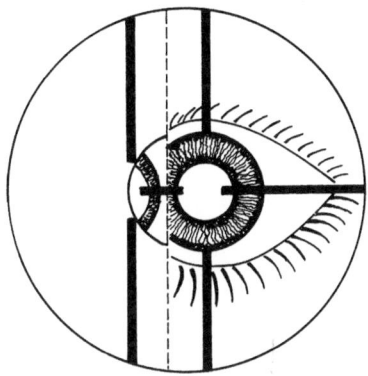

Fig. 25. View through the ocular with visualization of the corneal vertex in front and in profile

### 3.3.3 The Use of the Instrument

The governing attachment is connected with the house current and contains, in addition to an on-off button, a digital indicator for force exerted in a range of 0 to $1100 \times 10^{-5}$ N.

The reset button allows a quick return to the zero position. This makes it possible to obtain new measurements quickly.

The handheld instrument itself has three buttons: one lies beneath the handle and initiates the measurement. It is triggered with the index finger (Fig. 26).

Two other buttons are indicated with + or − and lie next to each other on the upper side (Figs. 27 and 28) of the handle.

These two buttons allow a continuous increase or decrease of the exerted force. If a static measurement is desired, the appropriate force is preset and the measurement is initiated by pushing the lower button.

This instrument, however, also allows dynamic measurements of corneal sensitivity. This is in contrast to all previous esthesiometers. The test body is advanced to the cornea with a preset subliminal force until contact is established. Only then will the force be increased continually by pushing the +/− button until the patient indicates

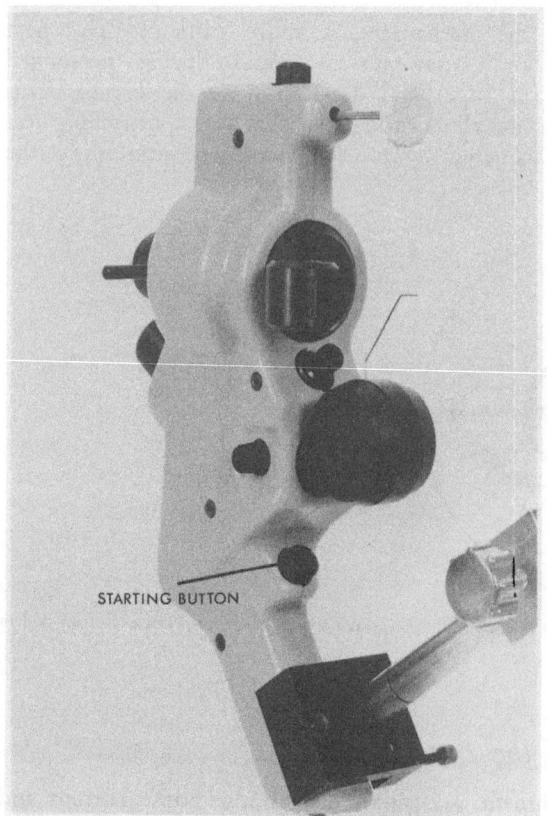

STARTING BUTTON

Fig. 26. Activating the release button

sensatio. The nonlinear increase of the exerted force is here of advantage as it shortens the time necessary for the measurement.

### 3.3.4 Technical Data of the Esthesiometer

Electrical current: 220 V/50 Hz, 0.2 A
Mechanical data when touching the cornea:
Range of force of the test body: maximally 10 mN $= 1000 \times 10^{-5}$N
Digital indication of the exerted force: 0 to $1000 \times 10^{-5}$N
Accuracy of the measurements of the force:

| Range of force | Maximal error |
|---|---|
| 0 ... 100 $\times 10^{-5}$N | 3 $\times 10^{-5}$N |
| 100 ... 1000 $\times 10^{-5}$N | 5 $\times 10^{-5}$N |

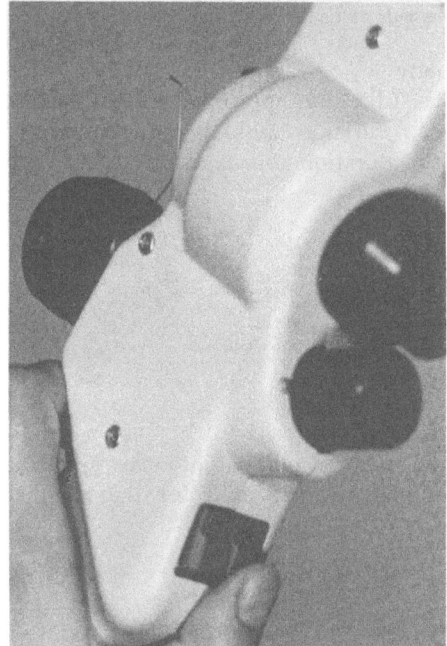

Fig. 27. Push button to regulate the force of the esthesiometer increase

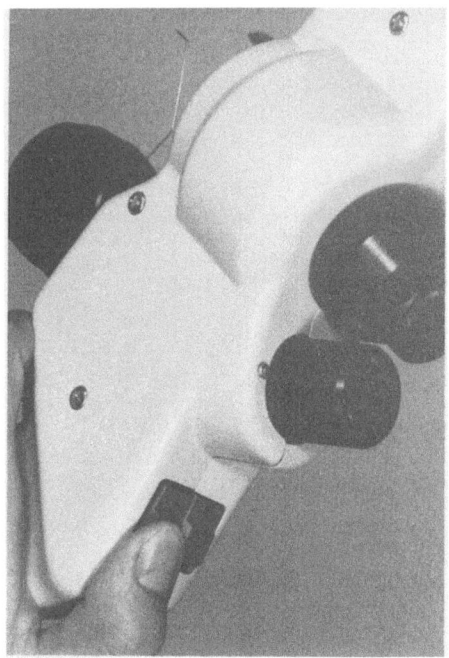

Fig. 28. Push button to regulate the force of the esthesiometer decrease

Speed of advancing the test body:
Fast speed:          7.7 mm/sec. (duration approximately 0.7 second)
Slow speed:          0.9 mm/sec. (duration approximately 0.6 second)
Reverse speed:       7.7 mm/sec. (duration approximately 1.4 seconds)
Observation microscope
Magnification
Main image:      5 ×
Lateral image:   5 ×
Exit pupil:
Location:            34 mm in front of the ocular
Diameter:            1.7 mm
Illumination:
Oblique illumination: 1 W
Sterilization: The handheld instrument is put into the automatic ultraviolet sterilization box similar to that used for the handheld applanation tonometer.

# 4. How to Use the Esthesiometer

The procedure should first be briefly explained to the patient. We suggest that the following points be discussed:

1. The various sensations which are produced by the measurements should be briefly described: heat, cold, tickling sensations, irritations and the sensation of touch.
2. It should be emphasized that even the slightest sensation should be indicated. (We frequently use the comparison that "even the sensation of a fine stream of air which passes the eye" should be indicated. To illustrate this point the skin of the hand can be gently touched with a piece of gauze.)
3. It has to be emphasized that no painful sensation should be expected. After such an explanation it is rare to find patients who are so apprehensive that their defense reflexes would make measurements difficult. (Similar conditions exist for applanation tonometry.)

The patient is comfortably seated on the stool and the head is placed against the adjustable neck rest (Fig. 29).

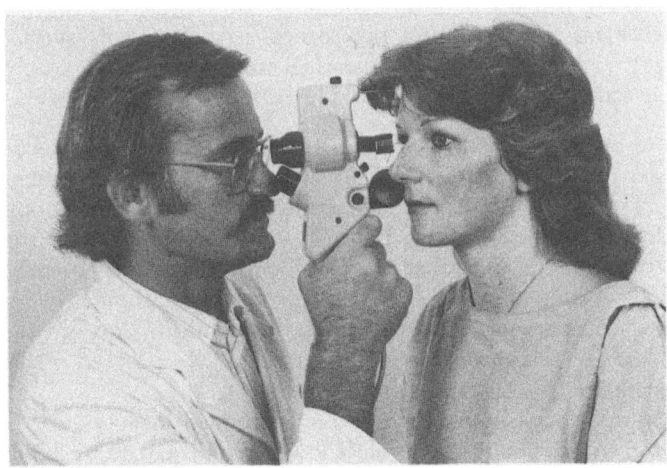

Fig. 29. Patient and examiner during a measurement

Without this neck rest, the patient may occasionally move his head during the procedure backward. A reasonably comfortable position of the patient will also avoid any uncomfortable positioning of the examiner. Patient and examiner are facing each other, somewhat laterally displaced, the knees are parallel to each other, the head of the examiner should be somewhat higher than that of the patient. During the entire time of the measurement, the patient and the examiner should be in a reasonably comfortable position in order to avoid any tension. The examiner (provided he is right-handed) holds the instrument in his right hand when examining the right or the left eye. The examiner should be able to use both his eyes for viewing.

The instrument is held in such a way that the thumb can easily push the buttons which change the exerted force while the index finger rests on the on-off button at the lower surface of the handle. The apparatus is now slowly approximated to the patient's eye in an oblique direction and guided by the examiner's eye. The front support is maximally extended and applied to the superior orbital margin in the area of the brows. The mirror tubes for the lateral observation is flipped temporally. The correct distance from the patient is obtained with the help of the reticule in the ocular. This should tangentially touch the corneal vertex. The examiner should, of course, maintain the optimal distance of the exit pupil. In this distance the main image and the lateral mirror image of the corneal profile are easily seen simultaneously. This observation in two planes allows us to:

1. direct the test body toward the desired area of impact;
2. maintain the correct distance of the instrument so that the impact of the test object will occur during the phase of slow advancement.
3. The test object will encounter the cornea vertically to its surface avoiding any shearing forces or shearing movements;
4. control exactly the time of impact (Fig. 30).

The other hand of the physician can gently keep the patient's lids apart in order to avoid the test body touching the lashes. The patient has to look into a desired direction in order to obtain a measurement on a specific area (if necessary, with the help of a fixation point in the examining room). If the corneal center is to be measured, the patient is asked to look "straight ahead," if the measurement should be at 3:00 o'clock he has asked to look "toward the right" or "toward the left" etc. Then the actual measurement can begin. We proceed in the following manner:

The measurement is initiated for a predetermined location with a subliminal force which should be well below the anticipated threshold. If the patient does not feel any sensation, the test body is pulled back and the force somewhat increased. The measurement can then be repeated. This has to be done until the patient for the first time notices a touch sensation. After the threshold has been approximately determined, the precise determination is obtained by bracketing the value from above and from below. If the patient gives reliable answers the threshold values are logged. If possible, the individual measurements should be accompanied by a definite supra and subliminal value. We accept as sensation response only the answer by the patient and not the lid reflex which is difficult to differentiate from the physiologic blinking.

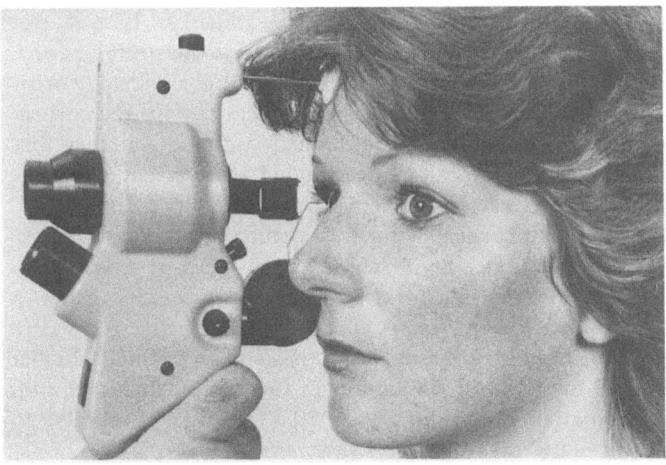

Fig. 30. The head of the patient rests against a neck support, the esthesiometer is in the correct position to perform measurements

During the measurement the following points have to be considered:

1. Touching of the lids and the lashes has to be avoided as this could lead to erroneous results.
2. A tremor of the examiner's hand and of the instrument or eye movements by the patient will lead to a shearing of the test object on the cornea and therefore to erroneous values. The time of impact should therefore be as short as possible.
3. Drying of the cornea induces an increase of the threshold (Cochet and Bonnet, 1969). The patient should close his eyes after every second or third measurement.
4. At certain intervals the surface of the test body has to be checked whether it is still black. If it begins to glisten it could irritate the patient.

# 5. Comparison Between Static and Dynamic Esthesiometry

The new electronic optical handheld esthesiometer makes it for the first time possible to perform a "dynamic" esthesiometry. Is was not possible with any of the previous instruments to raise the stimulus force continuously during corneal contact. This new method avoids any error due to the speed with which the test body advances toward the cornea. The instrument is advanced with a subliminal stimulus and therefore the threshold for touch alone can be determined. This is made possible by the very quick but exactly defined speed with which the exerted force increases. The first corneal contact is established with a subliminal stimulus which is then increased step by step until a sensation is perceived. This method is in contrast to the static esthesiometry in which a predetermined fixed force is applied to the cornea. As was to be expected, the threshold for dynamic esthesiometry is much higher than for the static method. At the limbus in the 6:00 o'clock position, the value for dynamic esthesiometry is $60.5 \times 10^{-5} \mathrm{N}$ compared to $21 \times 10^{-5} \mathrm{N}$ with static measurements (Fig. 31).

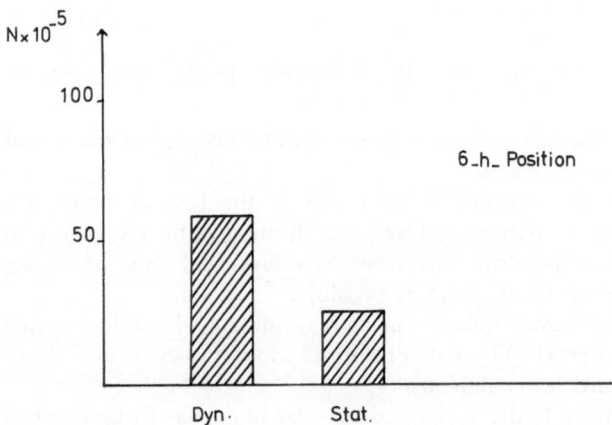

Fig. 31. Comparison of the thresholds for static and dynamic measurements (6:00 o'clock position)

This considerable difference in thresholds may be due to the fact that the increment in force occurs gradually and that any ballistic effect has been avoided. The latter was heretofore an uncontrollable variant which differed from instrument to instrument and from observer to observer. The advancement of the test body proceeds in our instrument with a precisely defined slow speed. This could, however, induce a different source of errors. We have to consider here the reaction time of the patient and of the examiner. These could retard the answers and thereby produce apparent higher threshold values. The patient can now interrupt with a simple switch any further increase of the applied force. This eliminates the reaction time of the observer altogether and shortens that of the patient. This improvement simplifies dynamic esthesiometry and facilitates its use of this method for clinical purposes.

# 6. *Topography of Corneal Sensitivity*

It was absolutely mandatory to establish an exact profile of corneal sensitivity in order to appreciate the results of clinical measurements. Only this would allow us to evaluate clinical problems of threshold changes. We therefore measured the corneal sensitivity at thirteen different areas of 20 to 40 year-old subjects. The measurements were taken on four meridians, at the limbus, 1 mm from the limbus, at a point between the center and this area, and at the center. These thresholds can be plotted as a characteristic profile (Fig. 32).

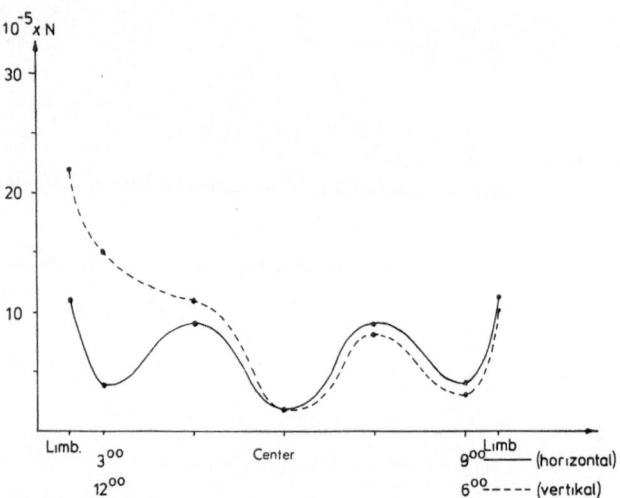

Fig. 32. Profile of corneal sensitivity (subjects between the ages of 20 to 40 years)

The lowest threshold lies at the corneal center and is lower than $1.0 \times 10^{-5}$ N. The threshold decreases in all four meridians to the next measured area up to $10.0 \times 10^{-5}$ N. Surprisingly, the thresholds decrease again at points 1 mm from the limbus in the nasal, temporal and lower periphery. The sensitivity decreases rapidly at the limbus.

Only the upper meridian differs from this behavior. The threshold value increases here gradually and continuously from the center toward the limbus. Theoretically, this may represent a neuronal adaptation to the continuous pressure by the upper tarsus.

# 7. The Receptor Field
## of Corneal Sensitivity

The amount of pressure necessary to reach a threshold is dependent from the size of the target. We therefore have to assume that there is a receptor field which has spatial dimensions and determines the threshold. If we assume that a force exerted on a surface can only produce pressure, then the established constant of a threshold equals the constant product of pressure times area, i.e. with increased area of touch a smaller pressure will be needed to reach threshold as more receptors will be stimulated.

We prepared nine plastic test bodies of different area size into which linen threads of varying rigidity were incorporated. The corneal sensitivity was then tested in the center and at the limbus while the subject was lying down. These targets represent test bodies of varying pressure and area. We did not establish thresholds for the individual test bodies and did not aim to grade the sensitivity. We only evaluated changes in sensitivity between the same subjects (similar to Marx, 1925). The number of subjects in which a definite test body could elicit a sensation was correlated to the total number of subjects tested. This was then expressed as percentage. The sensitivity tested in that way depends neither on the pressure ($r = -0.368$; $t = 0.887$; n.s.) nor on the force as the product of pressure times area ($r = 0.124$; $t = 0.281$, n.s.). On the other hand, the relation between sensitivity and the area of the test body is statistically significant ($r = 0.88$; $t = 4.149$; $0.005 < p < 0.01$). An even more significant correlation could be found between sensitivity and the product of area squared times pressure ($r = 0.965$; $t = 8.321$; $p < 0.0025$). Similar conditions exist at the limbus at 6:00 o'clock (Fig. 33).

As far as sensation is concerned, there is therefore an obvious dominance of area compared to pressure. This is just the opposite of what one would have expected. This allows certain conclusions as to the processing of the sensory excitation in the cornea. As the distance between corneal receptors, i.e. the free nerve terminations, is only 10 microns (Mensher, 1974), it would be impossible for the test object to hit an area without any receptor at all. The influence of the excited

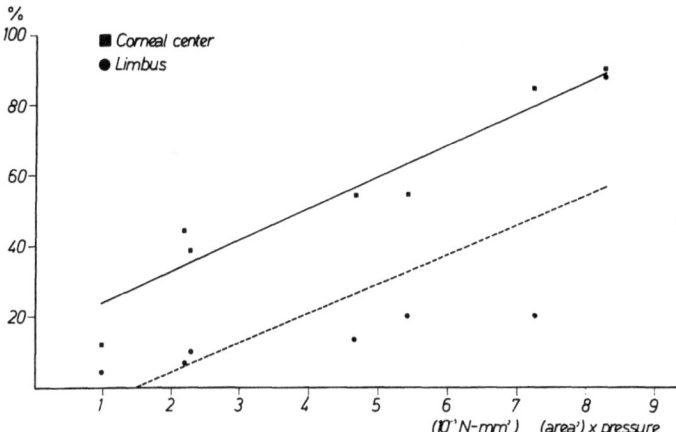

Fig. 33. The sensitivity is in direct relationship to the area squared times pressure. Ordinate: Subjects who perceived the stimulus expressed as percentage of the total number or subjects. Abscissa: Area squared times pressure in $10^{-5}$ N × mm²

area therefore means that the number of receptors stimulated is of utmost importance. The receptors or their afferent nerves form receptor fields. This additive spatial effect means that the action potential transmitted by one single receptor does not suffice to elicit a sensation.

# 8. Stimulus-Sensation – Relationship in the Cornea

Sensitivity thresholds alone give little information about the quality of sensation and they say nothing about the intensity felt by the patients. Therefore we carried out the following series of experiments with the new esthesiometer:

To determine the correlation between stimulus strength and sensation, six different forces ($1.5 - 3 - 6 - 12 - 24 - 48 \times 10^{-5}$N) were applied in a random sequence. Points of measurement were the corneal center and the limbus at 6:00 o'clock, one mm inside the cornea. Seven subjects were asked to classify the stimuli as "no feeling," "very weak," "moderate," "strong" and "very strong" without any previous training. They compared and classified the stimuli only according to their experience.

For statistical analysis the $\chi^2$-test and the Wilcoxon-test were used.

## 8.1 Results

### 8.1.1 Quality of Sensation

Over the whole range of stimulus intensity from 1.5 to $48 \times 10^{-5}$N all subjects only reported the sensation "touch." But this turned into the sensation "pain" when the stimulus remained in position for more than 1 sec. This holds true even for the smallest stimulus used. Only in one of the five examined subjects did the lowest stimulus ($1.5 \times 10^{-5}$N) not produce a sensation of "pain," even after a longer period of time. This subject suffered from an epidemic keratoconjunctivitis one year ago.

### 8.1.2 Graduation of Sensation

In the corneal center the smallest stimulus used ($1.5 \times 10^{-5}$N) is above the threshold in 13 out of 14 eyes. Thus, the highest stimulus used ($48 \times 10^{-5}$N) exceeds the threshold by a factor of thirty. At the limbus even stimuli of $12 \times 10^{-5}$N and more sometimes remain subliminal.

In short time applications of stimuli the perception is related to the sensation "touch." In Fig. 34 the degree of grayness represents the intensity of sensation. All subjects but one were able to discriminate between different stimulus strength, though sometimes the smallest stimulus used was felt more intensive than the strongest one. This held true for the center as well as for the limbus.

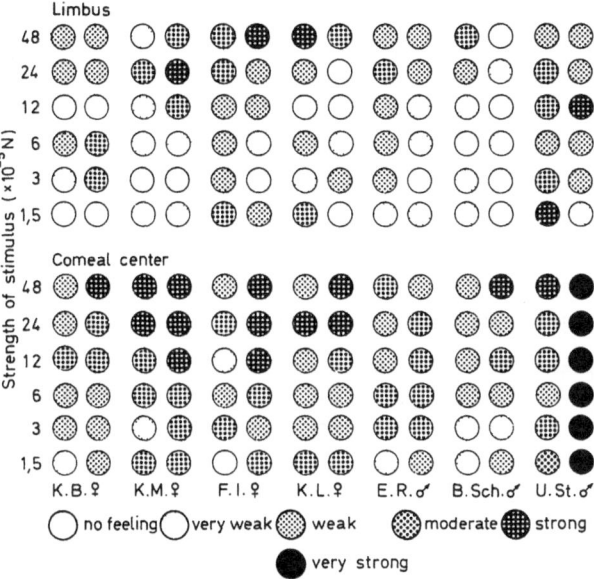

Fig. 34. Classification of stimulus strength (n = 7)

Only in a few eyes did the strength of sensation increase fairly proportionally with increasing stimulus intensity.

Fig. 35 illustrates how the sensation classification correlates with the different intensities in the corneal center. The smallest stimulus is preferentially classified as "very weak," "weak" and "moderate" whereas the strongest stimulus is frequently classified as "moderate" and "strong." "Very strong" was chosen by only one subject (U. St.) for all stimuli tested. This remarkable difference with the other eyes occurred only in the center. At the limbus his classification was similar to the other subjects. In spite of this special case, the different distributions of the six classification groups is statistically significant ($\chi^2$-test, $0.02 < p < 0.05$). An ever better significance is obtained in comparing only the classifications of the lowest ($1.5 \times 10^{-5}$N) and the highest ($48 \times 10^{-5}$N) stimulus with the Wilcoxon-test ($0.001 < p < 0.01$).

Corneal Center

| classification of sensation | 1,5 | 3 | 6 | 12 | 24 | 48 |
|---|---|---|---|---|---|---|
| very strong | X | X | X | X | X | X |
| strong | | | | X X | XXXXX | X X X XXXX |
| moderate | X X X X X X | XXXXX | XXXXX | X X X XXXX | XXXXX | X |
| weak | X X X | XXXXX | XXXX XXXX | X X X | XXXX | XXXX |
| very weak | XXX | XXX | | X | | X |
| no | X | | | | | |

Strength of stimuli $(10^{-3}N)$

$\chi^2 = 39.75$  $0.02 < p < 0.05$

Fig. 35. Distribution of stimulus strength to the different classes in the corneal center. Note: There is no rational scala

Limbus

| classification of sensation | 1,5 | 3 | 6 | 12 | 24 | 48 |
|---|---|---|---|---|---|---|
| very strong | | | | | | |
| strong | X | | | X | X | X X |
| moderate | X X | X X | X | X X | XXXX | XXXX |
| weak | X | XXXX | X X X X X X | X X X | X X X XXXX | X X X X X X |
| very weak | X X X X X X | X X X X X | X X X X X X | X X X | X | X |
| no | XXXX | X X X | X | XXXXX | X | X |

Strength of stimuli $(10^{-3}N)$

$\chi^2 > 25,58$  $p > 0,2$

Fig. 36. Distribution of stimulus strength to the different classes at the limbus

| classification of sensation | 1,5 | 3 | 6 | 12 | 24 | 48 |
|---|---|---|---|---|---|---|
| very strong | | X" | | | | |
| strong | | | | | X | X |
| moderate | | | | X X X | X | |
| weak | X | | X X | | | X |
| very weak | X | X X | | | | |
| no feeling | | | | | | |

Stimulus strength $(10^{-3}N)$

Fig. 37. Distribution of the first stimulus of each series to the different classes

At the limbus (Fig. 36) the sensation groups were not associated significantly with the stimulus strength ($\chi^2$-test, p > 0.05). The comparison between the classification of the lowest and the highest stimulus gave a worse significance at the limbus compared to the corneal center (Wilcoxon-test, 0.01 < p < 0.05).

Fig. 37 gives the classification of sensation to only the first stimulus of each series. The subjects chose nearly the same sensation groups for a definite stimulus as they did throughout the whole series. This seems to prove that the scale of sensations was established on a scale not biased by any comparison with a preceding stimulus.

## 8.2. Discussion

Our results show clearly at least two different kids of sensation on the cornea. Thus, they confirm the findings of Lele and Weddell (1956). The discrepancy between the observations and conclusions of Lele and Weddell on one side and of v. Frey and Strughold (1926) on the other may possibly be due to the continuance of the stimulus application. As shown in our own experiments, the discrimination between the sensation "touch," and "pain" is not really a matter of stimulus strength, but rather of the period of time the stimulus is applied. It would be difficult to touch the cornea for a definite short period of time by a handheld stimulus. This is possible, however, with the new esthesiometer because releasing the starting button takes the stimulus away from the cornea. But this instrument does not yet possess a defined timer. Thus, it is yet impossible to measure exactly whether a strong stimulus produces pain in a shorter period of time than a weak one. In all subjects a stimulus stronger than 30 times the threshold needs about a second to produce pain. And even a stimulus near the threshold causes pain after 1 to 2 seconds of application.

Two explanations seem to be possible: 1. Temporal summation in only one kind of nervous endings or channels makes the sensation turn from touch to pain. 2. There are at least two kinds of sensory endings in the cornea, one for touch and one for pain. Compared to other regions of the body both kinds of sensation show here approximately the same threshold. The pain sensation arises a little later. This explanation agrees with the histological findings that the cornea is supplied by C- and a-fibers (Zander and Weddell, 1951). The thinner fibers are found in the epithelium and the thicker ones on the stroma (Hoyes and Barber, 1976). The separation between "touch" and "pain" is also confirmed by single fiber recordings from the isolated cornea (Mark and Maurice, 1977) showing different sensory units for "pain" and "touch." Further insight may still be expected by measuring evoked potentials, though this is difficult and requires precisely reproducible stimuli. These can now be provided by the new esthesiometer.

The classification of stimulus strength on the cornea is rather vague (Fig. 34), but it seems to be more likely true scale than only a result of contrast obtained by previous comparison. Otherwise, it would be impossible to classify the first stimulus of a series. But even this stimulus can be discriminated according to its strength (Fig. 37).

At the limbus the classification is not as precise as in the center. This is not a fundamental difference, but rather results from the higher thresholds in this region: Near the threshold (corneal center) the ability to discriminate the stimulus strength is obviously more difficult (Figs. 35 and 36).

In the sensory organs we should expect a strict correlation between the intensity of the stimuli and the power applied. Bromm and Treede (1980) found the exponent of the power-pain correlation nearly at one. Thus, the strength sensation would be transformed linearly. Although in our experiments only a "touch" sensation is felt a linear transformation could still be possible proving the close relation between these two kinds of sensation, "touch" and "pain."

Finally, we could with the new esthesiometer show that the cornea has the ability of classifying the strength of a stimulus according to a scale and of discriminating between the sensation "touch" and "pain" if the stimulus is applied long enough.

# 9. The Sensitivity of the Conjunctiva

It has been known for a long time that similar to the cornea the conjunctiva possesses less discrimination between various stimuli than the skin. According to v. Frey and Strughold (1926) only touch and pain sensations can be elicited from the cornea; the conjunctiva has in addition a sensation for cold which we shall, however, not consider in this monograph. Previous authors (v. Frey and Strughold, 1926; Boberg-Ans, 1955; Norn, 1973) agreed that the threshold for touch sensation is in the conjunctiva considerably higher than in the cornea. The authors also agreed that there are regional differences. Especially in the horizontal meridian the differences in the thresholds may reach 100–200%; the higher thresholds are found close to the limbus; the lower ones in the nasal or temporal periphery (v. Frey and Strughold, 1926). Norn (1973) did not examine many conjunctival points, but his results also reflect a certain regional variability in the thresholds. The various authors, however, found different absolute values for these thresholds which probably is due to the variety of examination methods used (compare also Norn, 1976). v. Frey and Strughold (1926) found that the threshold of the conjunctiva (30 g/mm²) was 150 times higher than the threshold of the cornea (0.2 g/mm²), whereas Norn (1976) found that the conjunctival threshold (8.48 g/mm²) was only 8 times higher than that of the cornea (1.06 g/mm²). It should be emphasized, however, that in the latter publication the threshold was determined with the apparatus of Boberg-Ans or of Cochet-Bonnet and with these methods the corneal threshold is nearly identical with the smallest pressure which can be exerted. It is therefore possible that the values found are determined by the method used, especially since Boberg-Ans notes in his 1955 publication that the corneal thresholds were "<." This sign is missing in the later publications. We tried the Cochet-Bonnet apparatus on the conjunctiva of young subjects and were not able to exert pressure which would be subliminal. The new electronic handheld esthesiometer allows us to determine the conjunctival threshold as exactly as that of the cornea. The mean values and the ranges of the thresholds are shown in Fig. 38. They were determined on 20 eyes of 10 normal subjects with an age range from 20 to 50 years. The hatched areas show that the conjunctiva can be divided into different regions. The highest sensitivity was found in the conjunctiva near the temporal limbus. There are considerable differences when comparing this value with that found nasally above and below. The lowest sensitivity in the nasal conjunctiva is found in those parts of the upper and lower bulbar conjunctiva which are normally covered by the lids.

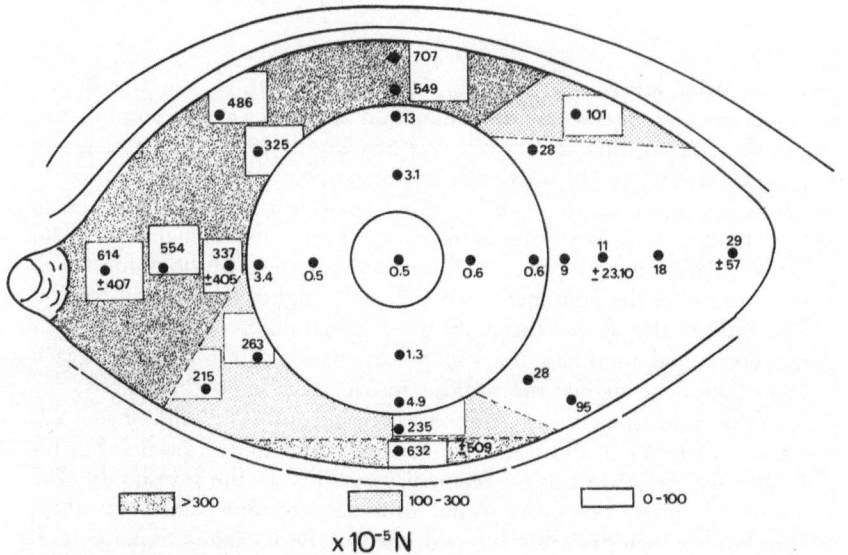

Fig. 38. Average thresholds of conjunctival sensitivity. The hatched areas represent different sensitivity

The large variations of the thresholds shown in Fig. 38 are probably not so much due to differences among the subjects, but due to the regional differences in the conjunctival sensitivity. Similar to the behavior of the skin, we have to distinguish here points of higher from points of lower sensitivity. Fig. 39 shows the thresholds in an $0.2 \times 0.2$ cm$^2$ area which was examined carefully point for point. A shifting of the test body by only 0.5 mm may result in a change of sensitivity by one log unit. We find on the temporal side also points with high thresholds, similarly on the nasal side a few point with low thresholds. Whether we can call one area of the conjunctiva more sensitive than another depends very much on the chance of hitting points with a low threshold. Therefore we cannot compare the results of various authors except when the density of the points tested was very high. The same holds for follow-up examinations when changes in the conjunctival sensitivity are suspected.

This interesting finding of discrete, but different points of individual sensitivity can only be explained by careful histologic studies. It is possible that at points of low threshold the receptors lie superficially under the epithelium or that we are dealing here with receptors of high sensitivity to begin with. It is also possible that these differences in

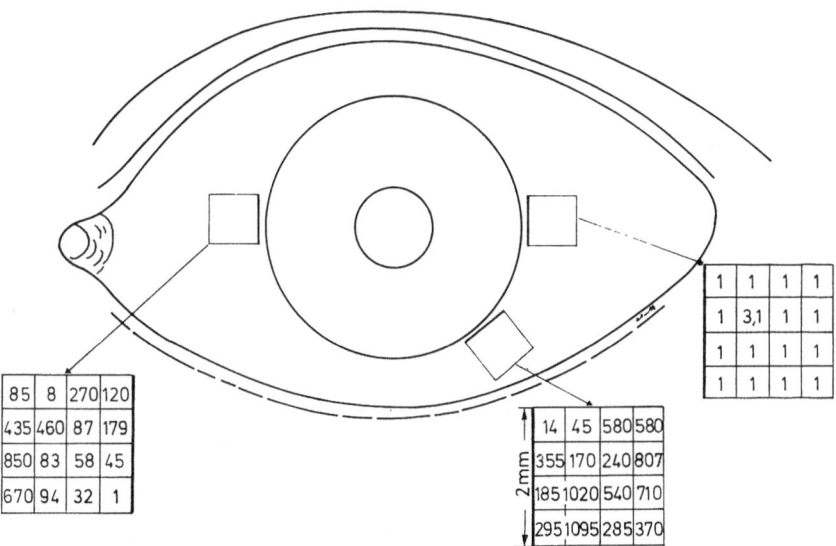

Fig. 39. Distribution of thresholds in a small conjunctival area

sensitivity may be due to a variable impedence by the epithelium or other tissues (compare also v. Frey and Strughold, 1926).

Schirmer (1963) reported that the threshold for tangential stimuli exerted with his spring esthesiometer on the cornea were lower than when the test body was approached from in front. Schirmer believes that this phenomenon is due to movement specific receptors. There is, however, an alternate explanation as far as the conjunctiva is concerned: The probability to hit a point of high sensitivity is higher when the test object is approached tangentially than when it is applied from in front. In order to test this hypothesis we determined the threshold for many points of a small square (Fig. 39), when the test body was approached radially (AP). Then the test body was applied to one of the sides of the square with a subliminal force. The subject now moves the eye slightly beneath the test body following a target so that the test object slides over a line in the previously examined square. This test is repeated

Table 1. *Comparison of the Thresholds With Anterior-Posterior (AP) and Tangential Application of the Stimulus; Area Size 2 × 2 mm²*

| Location* | nasal | nasal | nasal | nasal | nasal | nasal | nasal | nasal | temporal | temporal |
|---|---|---|---|---|---|---|---|---|---|---|
|  | 9 5 | 9 1 | 9 1 | 8 1 | 9 1 | 8 1 | 10 2 | 8 2 | 3 3 | 3 2 |
| Lowest threshold AP | 148 | 30 | 55 | 160 | 80 | 12 | 72 | 74 | 12.7 | 18 |
| Lowest threshold | 170 | 30 | 60 | 145 | 90 | 15 | 65 | 80 | 15 | 25 |

* First number: Position expressed in the meridian according to clock hours. Second number: Distance of the central margin of the area from the limbus.

several times while the test object is moved for a distance from the previous line corresponding to the width of its diameter. In that way all points of the tested square will be touched. We found in none of the subjects a threshold which was lower than the one found for the series of small points. Only when the threshold is increased will the subject feel the touch of the moving object (Table 1). We therefore have to conclude that the conjunctiva does not have any receptors differentiating between moving and static stimuli. The receptors react to a defined stimulus independent in which way it is applied.

# 10. The Localization of a Stimulus on Cornea and Conjunctiva

A stimulus can be evaluated not only for its quality and intensity but also for its location. We tested the ability to localize the stimulus under suprathreshold conditions on none fixed points. We tested eight subjects and the points were stimulated in a random sequence. The subject then drew on a large sketch of an eye the location of the point touched. In Fig. 40 the heavy symbols are the prechosen test points and the small symbols are the average response by the individual subjects. The deviations between the true location and the one indicated by the subject increase in horizontal direction from the center temporally and nasally; in general, the sensations are localized more peripherally than would correspond to the actual location. In the horizontal meridian significant error in localization occurred only close to the limbus in the points 5 and 7 of the conjunctiva. In the vertical meridian the deviation is usually upward and significant is only the erroneous localization of a stimulus in the center of the cornea.

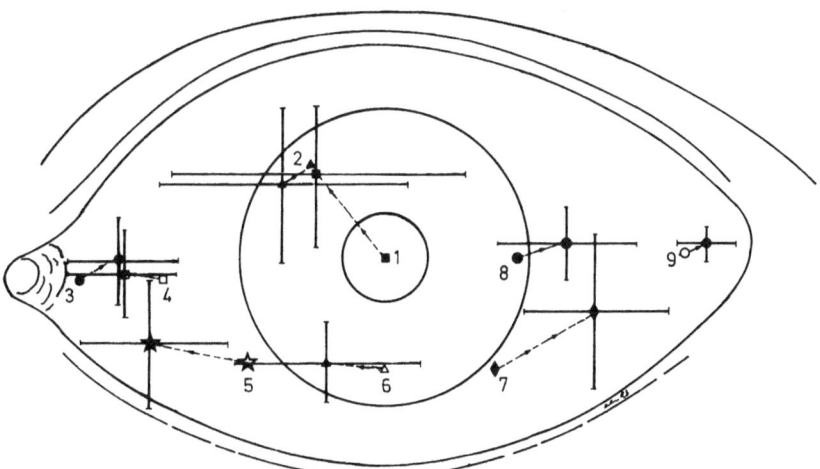

Fig. 40. Localization of a stimulus. The symbols without any variance signify the actual cite of the stimulus. The symbol with spread represent average values which the subject indicated as the site of excitation

The localization of stimuli is more accurate in the temporal and nasal canthi than in the cornea. This may be due to the central nervous connection from the receptors. The neural transmission from the cornea could contain more receptors than from a similar area of the conjunctiva. It is possible that the conjunctival receptors function like the corneal receptors not only as a defense mechanism, but may also help in recognizing the position of the eyeball within the palpebral fissure. For this purpose an unequivocal localization sense would be necessary.

# 11. The Lid Reflex as an Indicator of Corneal and Conjunctival Sensitivity

Some authors use the lid reflex as a measure of corneal sensitivity (Millodot, 1973; Gotz, 1972). This would only be valid if each touch which can be felt would also lead to a reflectory lid closure and if this reflex could not be voluntarily suppressed. A stimulus placed in the corneal center, even if it is slightly suprathreshold, will always elicit a reflectory lid closure. This reflex does not diminish or cease with repetition. We applied a series of five barely suprathreshold stimuli every two seconds. Each stimulus elicited a lid closure. When these series are repeated several times within a minute, the reflex is still undiminished. Subliminal thresholds will not lead to such a lid reflex.

The situation is different at the limbus. The lid reflex can be suppressed even if a considerably suprathreshold force of $400 \times 10^{-5}$N is used. Such a force will be felt as pain. The lid reflex is therefore only suitable for sensitivity testing at the corneal center.

# 12. The Age Dependency of the Corneal Sensitivity

It was necessary to investigate whether corneal sensitivity depends upon the patient's age. We have therefore measured the threshold at 6:00 o'clock in the corneal center and at 12:00 o'clock in groups of subjects varying between the ages of 20 to 40 years, 40 to 60 years and more than 60 years. The increase in threshold for the lower limbus and for the corneal center is small and insignificant even for persons older then 60. At 12:00 o'clock, however, the corneal sensitivity decreases to $30.0 \times 10^{-5}$N among the oldest subjects (Fig. 41).

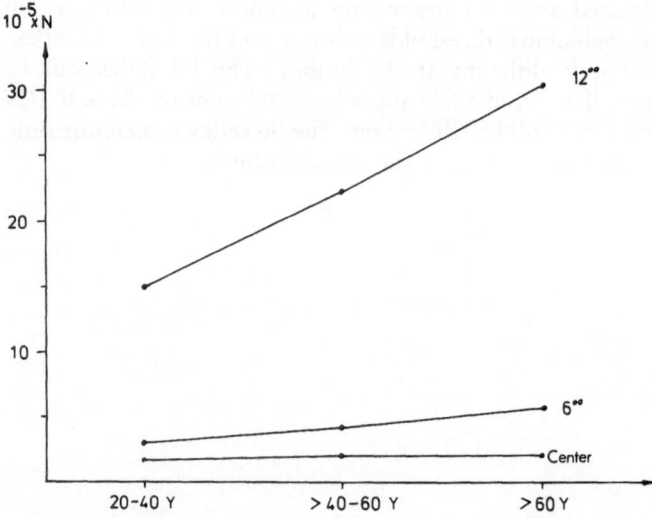

Fig. 41. Age dependency of corneal sensitivity

In a cornea with a senile arcus the lipid deposits will also cause a decrease of sensitivity (Forsius, 1958). Here again, the upper limbus is predominantly involved corresponding to the principal accumulation of these deposits (Velhagen, 1975). The sensitivity of patients with a sensile arcus is $201.5 \times 10^{-5}N$ compared to $32.5 \times 10^{-5}N$ among normal persons. This difference is less pronounced at the 6:00 o'clock meridian, but still significant with a value of $76.7 \times 10^{-5}N$.

# 13. Metabolic Influences on the Corneal Sensitivity

Previous investigators (Boberg-Ans, 1955) have attempted to study the metabolic influence on corneal sensitivity with inadequate methods. Cystine crystals or calcium deposits will decrease the sensitivity. A premature senile arcus in patient's with hyperlipidemia will also cause local sensitivity changes.

## 13.1 Corneal Sensitivity in Patients with Diabetes mellitus

Diabetes will involve nearly all tissues of the body. This may be due to a microangiopathy or to a polyneuropathy which may also involve the sensory innervation of the cornea (Downie *et al.*, 1961).

Schwarz (1974) made a thorough investigation on the effect of diabetes on corneal sensitivity; he compared the results in diabetic patients who were hospitalized with a group of normal persons and a group of diabetic patients who were treated as outpatients.

Using the esthesiometer of Cochet and Bonnet, he found no difference in corneal sensitivity between a group of diabetics who were inpatients and another group which was treated as outpatients; in addition, there was no correlation with age. On the other hand, corneal sensitivity decreased with increasing duration of the diabetes. There was also a significantly decreased corneal sensitivity among diabetic patients compared with the normal controls. Schwarz concluded that there was an axonal degeneration with segmental demyelinization leading to a distant neuropathy. Daubs (1975) also used the instrument of Cochet and Bonnet and comparing 30 diabetic patients with a control group, he found a significantly higher threshold for diabetics.

Nielsen (1978) investigated sensory sensitivity in diabetic patients in order to find a beginning polyneuropathy. For that purpose he examined not only corneal sensitivity, but also the sensory thresholds of other peripheral nerves. In a masked study, 36 diabetic patients were compared with a corresponding control group. The diabetics showed a significantly decreased sensitivity, but the sensitivity of peripheral nerves outside the cornea was reduced only in older patients. Nielsen did not consider the duration of the disease, the metabolic balance or the influence of treatment.

It seemed therefore indicated to investigate this clinical problem once again with the newer more precise examination methods. We wanted to find out whether the duration of the disease would influence corneal sensitivity; another question was the influence of the age of the patient or the mode of treatment. We also wanted to know whether there is a difference in the findings between juvenile and adult onset diabetes. Measurements were made at the corneal center and at the limbus at 6:00 o'clock. We also noted the time of the day when the examination was made, the sex of the patient and which eye had been examined.

We also noted the presence or absence of a rubeosis of the iris, the presence and severity of a diabetic retinopathy, of a cataract, of a poly-neuropathy and nephropathy. We examined in this way 183 eyes and compared them with 74 normal eyes of normal subjects of a similar age distribution.

We had 105 eyes of patients with juvenile diabetes and 78 cases of adult onset diabetes.

As far as the duration of the disease is concerned, we distinguished three groups:

1. a duration of less than five years,
2. a duration of five to ten years and
3. a duration of more then ten years.

We attempted to use the severity of a diabetic retinopathy as the yardstick of a microangiopathy in the eye. We therefore classified the fundus picture of our patients in the following way:

1. Thirty-three patients had no diabetic retinopathy.
2. A diabetic retinopathy was found in 45 patients (these were all patients with adult onset diabetes).

In order to evaluate the possible influence of the mode of therapy, we distingushed two groups of treatment:

1. Forty-five patients were only on oral medication.
2. Thirty-three patients were treated with insulin.

Our measurements were done at the limbus at 6:00 o'clock. The threshold values can be more precisely obtained at this area.

When comparing 105 juvenile diabetics with a normal population, we found a mean value of $12.2 \times 10^{-5} N$ in the diabetics and $4.6 \times 10^{-5} N$ among the healthy persons. The difference is highly significant with a $p <$ than 0.001 (U-test) Fig. 42).

Similar results were obtained in the group of older patients: the mean was among 78 diabetic patients $43.3 \times 10^{-5}N$ compared to $15.5 \times 10^{-5}N$ for the normal group (Fig. 42). The difference between the two groups is again significant with a $p <$ than 0.001.

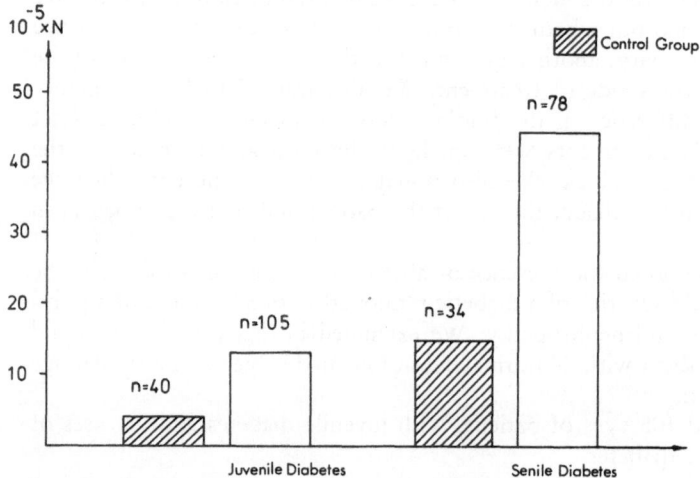

Fig. 42. A comparison of the corneal sensitivity among patients with juvenile or adult onset diabetes and a control group

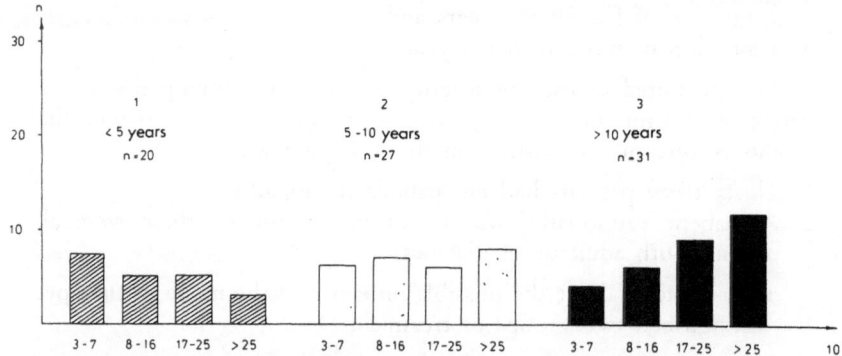

Fig. 43. Change of corneal sensitivity in relation to the duration of the diabetes

We then examined the relationship of corneal sensitivity to the duration of the diabetes. We shall discuss here only the adult onset diabetics (Fig. 43).

There is a statistically significant decrease of sensitivity with increasing duration of the disease: In the group of patients with the shortest duration of diabetes "normal" sensitivity predominates; in the next group, those patients who had diabetes for five to ten years, the frequency curve shows a peak at a considerably decreased threshold value. This difference becomes even more conspicuous when compared with patients who had the disease for more than ten years.

Results of the U-test:

U I/III = 2.447         p < 0.02,
U II/III = 2.0913      p < 0.05.

A statistically significant difference was also found when comparing 33 patients with normal fundus with 45 patients with a retinopathy (U = 2.06  p < 0.05). The number of patients with considerably increased threshold values is in the group with retinopathy considerably higher (Fig. 44).

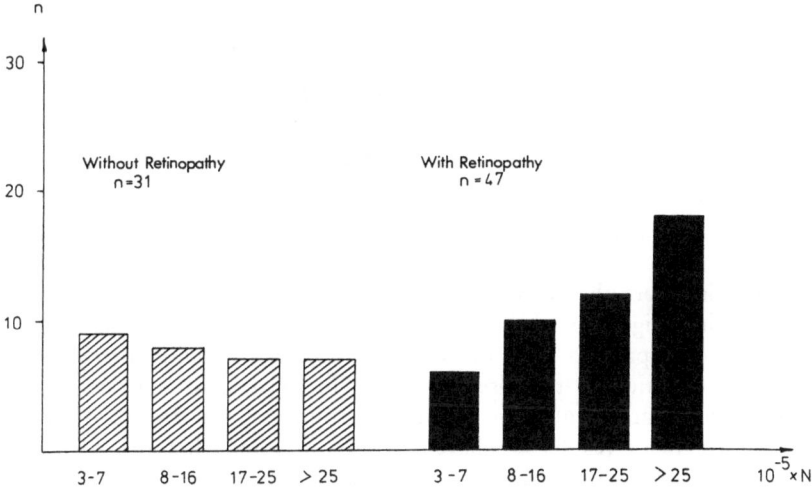

Fig. 44. Corneal sensitivity in patients with an adult onset diabetes with and without retinopathy

These results are practically identical with those obtained when comparing corneal sensitivity with the duration of diabetes. This affirms a widely held clinical impression. We generally expect in patients with adult onset diabetes a retinopathy only after the patient had the disease for at least ten years. It would be interesting to perform a multifactorial analysis of these results in order to differentiate the influence of the disease from morphologic fundus changes. Unfortunately, this was not possible in our series as the number of cases was too small.

Most interesting are the results obtained when comparing different modes of treatment. In general, it can be assumed that the majority of patients with adult onset diabetes is first treated with oral medication, whereas insulin will be used only at a later date. While we did find a correlation between corneal sensitivity decrease and duration of the disease, we could also show that patients on insulin had a lower threshold (Fig. 45).

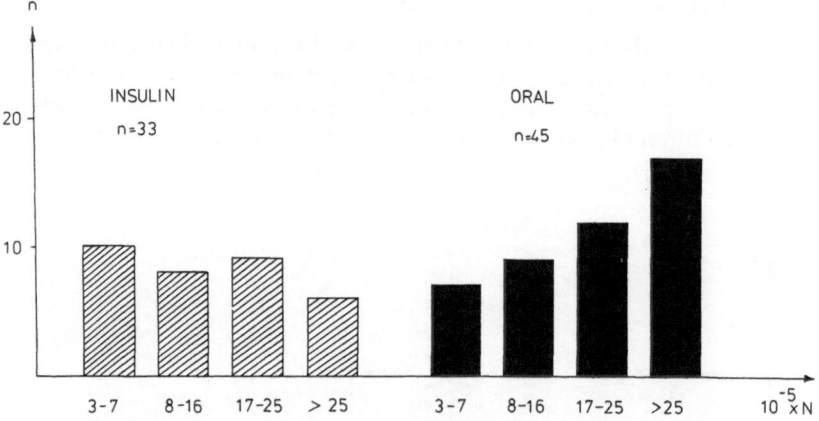

Fig. 45. Correlation between corneal sensitivity and mode of treatment

We find here that $U = 0.836$   $p < 0.5$.

Our investigations confirm previous results that corneal sensitivity is reduced in patients with diabetes. We found a definite correlation with the duration of the disease. This is in contrast to Schwarz, but probably in agreement with the clinical course of the disease. When evaluating these results we have to keep in mind that the corneal sensitivity decreases with age regardless of the disease state. Our patients with adult onset diabetes were usually patients of advanced age and therefore should have had decreased thresholds. Nevertheless, comparing this group of patients with an age adjusted group of normals, this difference is still significant.

As was to be expected thresholds among patients with retinopathy were significantly higher than among patients with a normal fundus.

It is remarkable that patients on insulin had a lower threshold than patients on oral medication. If we interpret the status of corneal sensitivity as an expression of morphologic conditions and damages, we could assume that patients on insulin are in a more advantageous metabolic balance. In order to prove this assumption, extensive studies with multifactorial analyses considering the age of the patient, the duration of the disease, the dosage of insulin and accompanying metabolic changes would be necessary.

We believe that measuring corneal sensitivity as a routine procedure for diabetic patients would help us to determine the further course of the disease; a change in corneal sensitivity may be an important indicator as to the prognosis and further progression.

From a general point of view the observed changes in threshold values may not be too important. The remaining corneal sensitivity still guarantees the detection of superficial corneal erosions or of a corneal foreign body. A clinical significance may exist for patients who wear contact lenses or suffer from an advanced stage of the disease.

## 13.2 Corneal Sensitivity After Light Coagulation

Light coagulation of diabetic retinopathy has become an important mode of treatment. Numerous reports have been published concerning the possible well-known complications of such a treatment, e.g. retinal or choroidal hemorrhages, loss of visual field, transient myopia, secondary vitreous changes, ischemic optic neuropathy, cystoid macular edema, or increased lens opacities. Another complications are associated pathologic changes of the cornea. A few report deal with damage to the ciliary nerves. Rogell (1979) reported eight eyes of juvenile diabetics with an internal ophthalmoplegia after argon laser coagulation. He explained this as a heat damage to the short parasympathetic fibers of the ciliary nerves.

It seemed reasonable to test this hypothesis by examining the corneal sensitivity after photocoagulation. We examined 37 diabetics between the ages of 21 and 80 who received photocoagulation for diabetic retinopathy. Among these were 11 patients with juvenile diabetes and 28 with an adult onset diabetes. A panretinal coagulation was performed on 27 eyes because of proliferative diabetic fundus changes; in 7 patients the panretinal coagulation was performed with the xenon light (Fankhauser attachment); 5 eyes received only focal laser coagulations because of an exudative maculopathy. The coagulation encompassed usually the entire nasal half of the fundus, while in the temporal half the retinal area within the vascular arcade remained untreated. We measured in 27 patients the corneal sensitivity before and after the treatment and in 10 patients only after the light coagulation had been applied. In patients who also had a preoperative examination the follow up extended up to six months; in patients who had only postoperative examinations the follow up extended up to four and a half years.

A statistical evaluation of the results showed a mean value of corneal sensitivity at the limbus at 6:00 o'clock of $18.0 \times 10^{-5}N$ after laser coagulation compared to a mean value of $8.0 \times 10^{-5}N$ before treatment (Fig. 46).

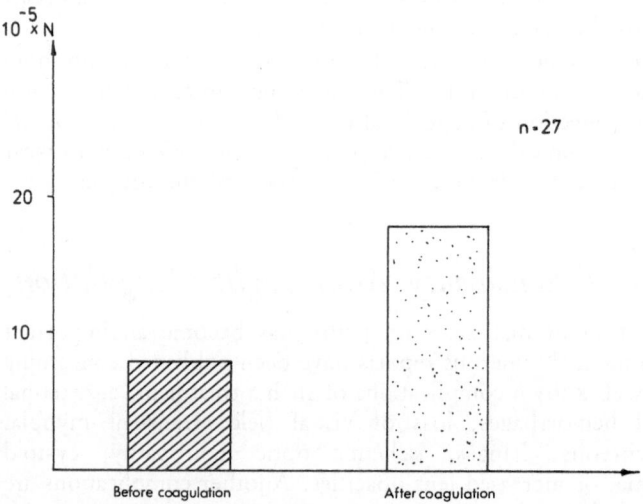

Fig. 46. Corneal sensitivity before and after argon laser coagulation, 27 patients

The difference is statistically significant with $U = 2.72$ $p < 0.01$.

If we now divide our patient material into various groups according to the mode of light coagulation, we find a mean value of the seven cases which were treated with the xenon light (Fankhauser attachment, three-mirror contact lens) of $27.5 \times 10^{-5}N$ compared to $18.0 \times 10^{-5}N$ for 27 patients treated with argon laser. This difference is also statistically significant with $U = 2.26$ $p < 0.05$ (Fig. 47).

We have to consider, however, that the two groups differed also in other aspects. In all cases argon laser coagulation we used surface anesthetics exclusively, whereas in xenon coagulation we added a retrobulbar injection. We therefore have to consider the theoretical influence of this injection on the sensitivity threshold (see also 14.4 on the influence of the mode of anesthesia on postoperative corneal sensitivity).

On the other hand, the marked difference of the values could be the effect of a generally stronger coagulation effect of the xenon coagulator; this applies especially to the size of the area treated. One could conclude that the decrease in corneal sensitivity is in direct proportion to the applied coagulation energy.

The decreased sensitivity after light coagulation is due to a thermal injury to the corneal nerves. This applies especially to the final branches of the long ciliary nerves which course in the epichoroidal space (Binder and Riss, 1981).

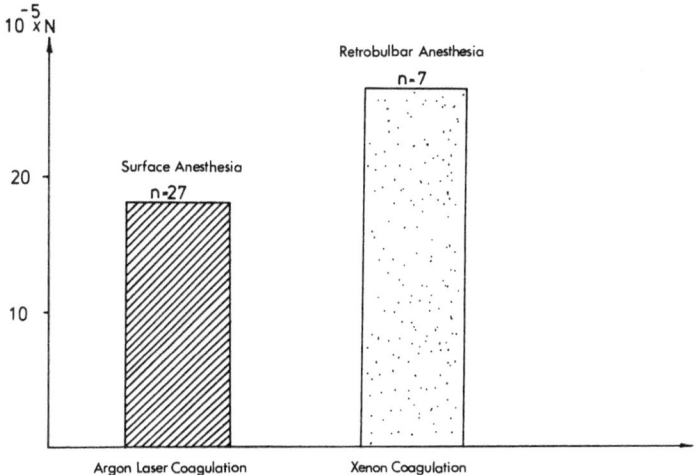

Fig. 47. Corneal sensitivity after xenon or laser coagulation (surface anesthesia with or without retrobulbar injection)

## 13.3 Changes in Corneal Sensitivity During Pregnancy

Numerous authors have examined the many metabolic changes occurring during pregnancy. The eye becomes hypotonic (Millodot, 1977); changes in the visual fields and a "myopia of pregnancy" have been described.

Millodot (1977) found changes of corneal sensitivity in women during the last weeks of pregnancy. Similar changes have been described with menstruation. There was a slow, but continuous increase of the thresholds from the 12th week of pregnancy to delivery. After the 31st week of pregnancy, these values were significantly lower than in a control group. The original values were reached six to eight weeks after delivery. Millodot believed that this was due to a general water retention during pregnancy as the difference was especially pronounced in women who were overweight or had edema of the ankles and the fingers.

We tried to reinvestigate this question with the new more precise instrument.

We examined 86 women between the 13th and 40th week of pregnancy. Their mean age was 25.3 years. All women were examined for signs or symptoms of a toxemia (edema, proteinuria and a blood pressure higher than 135/85 mm Hg). Affected patients were classified according to the toxemia index of Goecke and Schwabe. Thirteen patients were myopic, one was a hyperope. The corneal sensitivity was measured at the limbus at 6:00 o'clock and, in general, both eyes were examined. As a control we measured 37 eyes of normal nonpregnant women. Their mean age was 25.8 years.

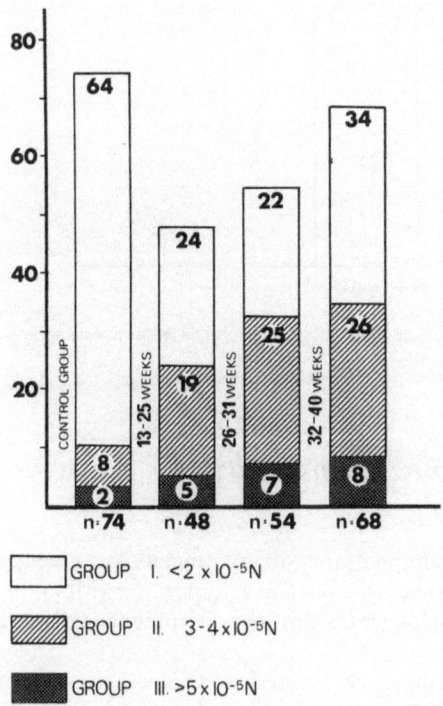

Fig. 48. Distribution of corneal sensitivity in pregnant and nonpregnant women

Among the 86 pregnant women 23 had symptoms of a mild toxemia (13 with a toxemia index of 1, 8 with an index of 2 and 1 women with an index of 3).

In order to evaluate changes of corneal sensitivity we divided our patients into three groups:

1. a corneal sensitivity of less than or equal to $2 \times 10^{-5}$N;
2. a corneal sensitivity between 3 and $4 \times 10^{-5}$N and
3. a corneal sensitivity higher than $5 \times 10^{-5}$N.

A number of pregnant women had during the last trimester of pregnancy a threshold between 8 and $10 \times 10^{-5}$N. Such thresholds were never found in the control group (Fig. 48).

The decreased corneal sensitivity among pregnant women was not related to the duration of the pregnancy.

In general, we found in this small sample a reduced corneal sensitivity among pregnant women compared to a control group (Riss and Riss, 1981).

# 14. The Effect of Surface Anesthetics

Surface anesthesia plays an increasingly important role in clinical ophthalmology. In the past it was mainly used for tonometry and the removal of corneal foreign bodies. Nowadays a number of diagnostic measures need surface anesthesia: the use of contact lenses for the examination of the fundus or the chamber angle would be impossible without the use of mild and quickly acting surface anesthetics. Electroretinography and echography also need a surface anesthesia of the cornea. The demand has increased for rapidly acting anesthetic agents which should be free of any side effects. This demand is mainly due to the increased need for glaucoma screening with the applanation tonometer.

A variety of medications have been put on the market by the pharmaceutical industry. The question has therefore arisen which one is the best for the needs of the ophthalmic practice.

Heretofore it was not possible to measure quantitatively the anesthetizing effect of such drugs. Nor could they be compared with each other.

This was due to the fact that a reliable reproducible measuring method was not available.

Marx compared in 1925, various local anesthetics in different concentrations concerning their effect on the cornea. He used a hair of 75 mg force and noted the number of perceived sensations in a test which consisted of 20 corneal contacts.

Emmerich, Carter, and Berens examined in 1955 the duration of anesthesia produced by Proparacain-Hydrochloride (Benoxinat). They used a fine cotton fiber and touched with it the corneal limbus. The clinical results varied considerably.

Linn and Vey (1955) used instead of the v. Frey hair nylon threads of varying rigidity. They did not find any difference in the duration of anesthesia produced by various local anesthetics.

Klingmüller (1957) tested the influence of the vehicle or solvent on the effect of a surface anesthetic on the rabbit eye. He also used hair for a stimulus.

The introduction of the quantitatively reproducible esthesiometer made it possible to test various surface anesthetics on the eye. A number of such medications are available. They differ in their concentration, buffer and basic chemical substance.

Mode of action:

A local anesthetic applied to the corneal surface diffuses into the tissue and accumulates in the membranes of the sensory nerve endings. It alters here several parts of the cell membrane closing the $Na^+$-pores. This ceases or decreases the irritability of the nerve (Strichartz, 1976). The sensitivity changes are inversely proportional to the effect of the applied anesthetic. The loss of sensitivity can be measured by determining the stimulus necessary to elicit touch sensation in the cornea.

The biologic effect of a superficial local anesthetic depends on several factors:

1. the composition and characteristics of the applied medication, e.g. its lipid solubility, electric charge, molecular weight and structure (Büchi et al., 1964; Ritchie and Cohen, 1975) (Fig. 49).

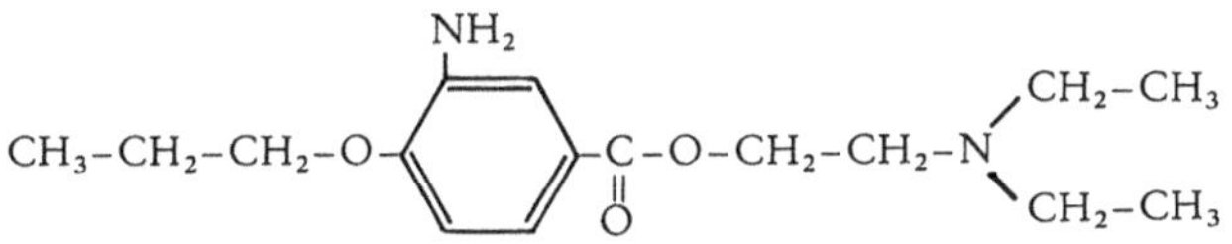

Fig. 49. Chemical structure of Proxymetacain

A typical local anesthetic contains a tertiary aminoradical which is through an intermediary chain (ester or acid amide) connected to an aromatic ring. The dissociation balance lies in relation to the pKa value between 80 and 90% of the conjugated acid. Only the small alkali moiety is capable of penetrating the tissue barriers. The molecular effect on the nerve membranes is due to the charged cation form of the tertiary aminoradical in which the nytrogen is quarternary (Kuschinsky and Lüllmann, 1976).

2. On the physical-chemical properties of the vehicle, especially of its pH value, and of the additives, e.g. preservatives and tensides (Ophthalmica, Vol. 1, 1975). Thoma (1977) demands a physiologic and chemical compatibility of all compounds contained in a medication with optimal effect under consideration of its tolerance, sterility and stability.

3. On the composition of the precorneal tear film (S. Ehlers, 1965; Rintelen, 1969; Rohen, 1977) as this represents the distribution

medium for the surface anesthetic (Ophthalmica, 1975). The administration of solutions with unphysiologic pH will strongly stimulate the lacrimal gland. The amount of the administered medication and the buffer capability of the tear fluid are also important for this reaction (Ophthalmica, 1975, page 82). These surface anesthetic hydrochloride compounds are prepared as an acid solution. Their optimal stability lies outside the irritation free tolerance margins (Trolle and Lassen, 1958; Moses and Cotlier, 1970).

4. On the histologic structure of the cornea (Busacca, 1963; Rohen, 1964; Duke-Elder, 1968; Moses and Cotlier, 1970). Lipid-containing barriers, e.g. the corneal epithelium and endothelium, are easily permeable to depolarized radicals in the dissociated form; water-containing tissues, e.g. the corneal stroma, are permeable for polarized dissociated radicals.

5. On the number and distribution of free nerve endings in the tissue.

We wanted to investigate in our experiments not only the various concentrations and modes of administration of local anesthetics, but also the influence of the vehicle (macromolecules, pH values). Clinical experience has shown that after the application of a surface anesthetic a more or less complete anesthesia of the cornea will rapidly set in. The duration of this anesthesia may vary. The recovery phase begins with a period of decreased corneal sensitivity. We performed some pilot studies on six subjects, but found that the loss of sensitivity occurred so rapidly that it was not possible to differentiate various medications even if the stimulus was quickly and rapidly increased. During the period of anesthesia, all surface anesthetics had the same effect and even a stimulus of $1000 \times 10^{-5}$ N did not elicit any sensation. Our comparisons of various medications had therefore to be done during the recovery phase. The medication is slowly broken down and absorbed. This will finally lead to a phase when the maximal stimulus, which had been subliminal during the anesthesia, will again be perceived as a sensation. This means that the pharmacological agent is being eliminated from the area of its effect, i.e. the nerve membranes. The further decrease in the effectiveness of the medication expresses itself as a decrease in thresholds for touch. We took as our index of comparison the time elasped between the administration of the anesthetic and the moment when a stimulus of defined strength will again just be perceived. Further investigations showed us which were the appropriate stimulus forces to obtain the best results for comparisons. We used four threshold values, i.e. 1000, 600, 200 and $1 \times 10^{-5}$ N. These forces proved to be most suitable and reproducible in measuring and comparing the duration of surface anesthetics.

In these pilot studies we also tried to determine the optimal time intervals between measurements. The first measurement was performed three minutes after the application of the anesthetic into the conjunctival sac. We used here a force of $1000 \times 10^{-5}$ N. This measurement was repeated every minute at the same area (corneal center) until the patient indicated a sensation of touch. In order to exclude any possible wrong responses, we repeated the experiment with the same stimulus force. Only when the second one was also perceived was the stimulus reduced and the next threshold determined. There is less frequent blinking under the influence of the anesthetic and we therefore asked the patients to close their eyes briefly after every contact with the test body. This avoided any drying of the epithelium. The administration of the anesthetic was standardized both in the amount applied and in the exact details of the application. We preferred the subjective response of the patient over the blink reflex as an indication whether the contact with the cornea was perceived or not. During the recovery phase, a stimulus may elicit the sensation of touch, but not yet provoke a blink reflex. We selected the patients carefully as the results depended upon their subjective responses. We first tested the normal corneal sensitivity of each person before the experiment was started. We also excluded any subject who indicated a reaction or intolerance to local anesthetics.

We did not consider the diurnal variations of corneal sensitivity as described by Millodot (1972). They are of too small an amplitude to influence our results. Our findings on the topographic distribution of corneal sensitivity (Draeger *et al.*, 1976) led us to choose the corneal center as the site of impact.

The statistical evaluation was made by variance analysis. This method is suitable for all problems in which various factors may contribute to the total distribution of data. It allows us to evaluate specifically those results which are relevant to our investigation. The following factors influence the experiment:

the pressure exerted,
the patient and
the topical medication.

Variance analysis allows us to differentiate these factors. By eliminating the factors, the exerted force and the examined patient, it was possible to measure and calculate quantitatively the influence of the anesthetics alone.

We examined the effect of various commercial preparations (Table 2).

Table 2. *Tested Medications, Their Concentrations, Dosage and pH Differences, as well as Their Preservatives*

| | |
|---|---|
| Proprietary preparation | Chibro® Kerakain<br>Novesine® 0.4%<br>Conjucain®<br><br>Fluorescein-Benoxinat Eye Drops<br>"Mann"<br>Thilorbin® |
| Concentration | 0.1% solution of Proxymetacain<br>0.5% solution of Proxymetacain<br>1.0% solution of Proxymetacain |
| Dosage | 1 drop of Chibro® Kerakain<br>2 drops of Chibro® Kerakain<br>3 drops of Chibro® Kerakain |
| Environment (pH) | Two drops of a borax solution are instilled into the eye in order to buffer the subsequent instillation of one drop of Chibro® Kerakain |
| Preservative | 0.5% solution of Proxymetacain with<br>a) Chlorbutanol (0.5%)<br>b) Chlorhexidin (0.01%)<br>c) Benzalkoniumchloride (0.01%) |

We also investigated the effect of three different concentrations of the anesthetic, the dose response curve, the influence of the pH and of the admixture of various preservatives (Draeger *et al.*, 1980).

*1. Commercial Preparations.* Nearly all the preparations contained as effective ingredient Oxybuprocain in a concentration of 0.4% (0.45% for fluorescein-benoxinat eye drops). The only exception was Chibro-Kerakain® (0.5% Proxymetacain).

In spite of a difference in composition of the vehicle (preservative, macromolecules, fluorescein as an additive), these anesthetics did not show any difference in the duration of their effect. Two preparations contained as an additive cellulose-ether (Conjucain® and Polyvidon®, fluorescein-benoxinat eye drops) in order to increase their viscosity. This did not prolong the duration of the anesthesia (Fig. 50).

*2. Concentration.* We investigated the relationship of the duration of the anesthesia with the concentration and dose of the anesthetic (dose response curve). We obtained the following results for Proxymetacain (INN) = Proparacaine hydrochloride (USP XIX):

The duration of the anesthetic effect increases with increasing concentrations of 0.1%, 0.5% and 1%. However, there is no linear relationship between the concentration and the duration of the effect (Fig. 51).

DIFFERENT PREPARATIONS

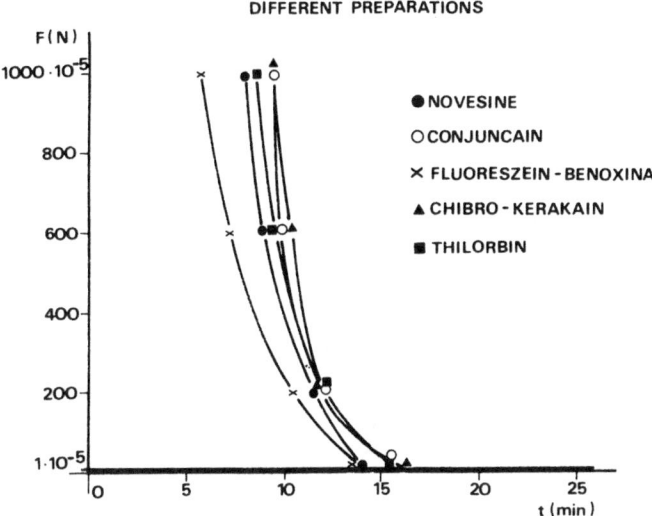

Fig. 50. Duration of the anesthetic effect of various commercial preparations

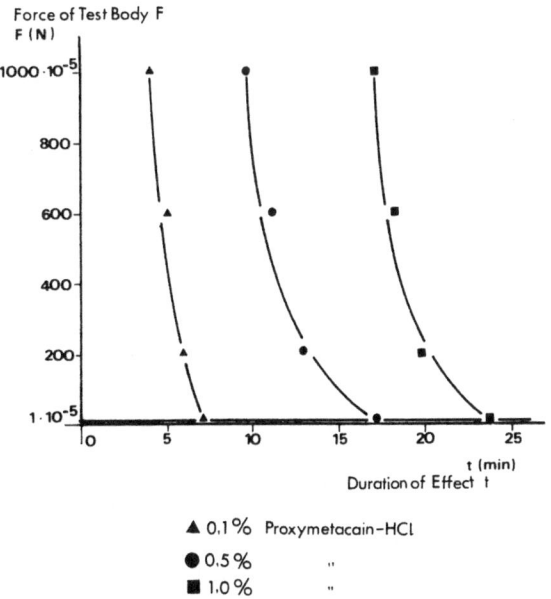

Fig. 51. Duration of the anesthesia when varying the concentration

6    Draeger et al., Corneal Sensitivity

3. *Dose.* The duration of the anesthesia varied with the dosage applied. This was established when 1, 2 or 3 drops of Chibro-Kerakain® were instilled (Fig. 52).

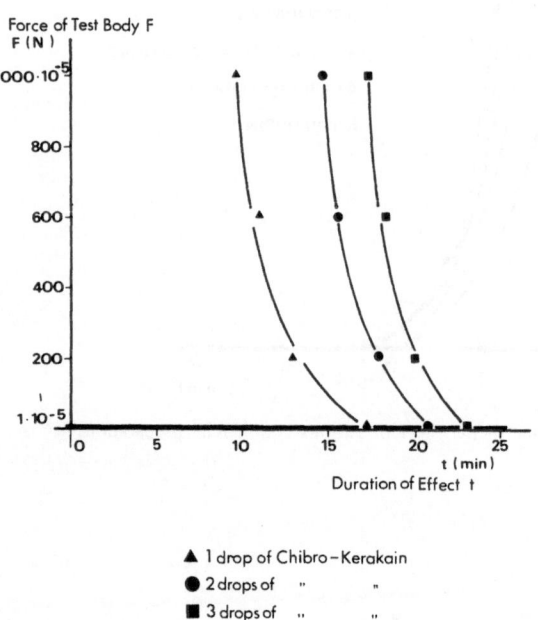

▲ 1 drop of Chibro–Kerakain
● 2 drops of   "       "
■ 3 drops of   "       "

Fig. 52. Duration of anesthesia when varying the dose (dose response curve). Anesthetic used: Chibro-Kerakain®

4. *Environment.* The composition of the precorneal tear film in which the surface anesthetic will be distributed influences, according to our experience, the duration of the anesthesia. If the corneal surface is first buffered with a 2.6% solution of borax (pH 9.2), the duration of the anesthesia was increased. If the precorneal tear film is made alkaline, then the effect of one drop of Chibro-Kerakain® equals the effect of two drops of Chibro-Kerakain® when no borax solution is given.

5. *Preservatives.* Evaluating the influence of preservatives on the effectiveness of an anesthetic gave the following results: The various preservatives (Benzalkonium-chloride 0.01%, Chlorbutanol 0.5% and Chlorhexidine 0.01%) added to an 0.5% solution of Proxymetacain did not influence the duration of the anesthesia when the usual modes of application and dosages were used.

## 14.1 Discussion of Our Results

*a) Comparison of the duration of anesthesia for five selected commercial preparations.* It seems remarkable that we did not find any differences in the duration of the effect among all the preparations examined, though two of them contained cellulose-ether or Polyvidon in order to increase their viscosity. We therefore can confirm the results obtained by Adriani (1964); he also did not find any significantly increased anesthesia when macromolecules were added. This finding, however, can not be extended to cover other liquid ocular medications.

Pilocarpine-hydrochloride shows an improved efficancy when hydrophilic macromolecules are added (Hardenberger, Hanna, Boyd, 1975). This difference in the effect of added macromolecules lies in our opinion in the different site of action of the medications. The distance which the local anesthetics have to travel in order to reach the end organs of the sensory nerves is too short to be influenced by improved adhesiveness.

*b) The influence of the concentration on the duration of the anesthesia.* This relationship between the duration of anesthesia and the concentration of the drug holds for those concentrations which do not damage the corneal epithelium.

*c) The influence of the dose upon the duration of the anesthesia.* There is certainly an influence of the dose upon the duration of the anesthesia, but this is limited by the capacity of the conjunctival sac and the excretory lacrimal system. The following result points towards such a relationship: When a certain volume of fluid is exceeded the conjunctival sac cannot hold it, nor can the lid blink guarantee an even distribution. The fluid will escape via the lacrimal system or will overflow at the palpebral margin.

*d) The influence of a borax solution on the duration of the anesthesia.* The influence of the environment upon the effect of a local anesthetic is well known. This applies not only to the vehicle in which the medication is used, but also to the tissue into which the medication penetrates. The pH influences the dissociation balance. In an inflamed tissue which shows a lower than normal pH (Kuschinsky and Lüllmann, 1976) the balance will be shifted toward the acid side. Less diffusible free base is available and the effectiveness of the local anesthetic decreases.

Our experiments have shown that it is possible to shift the dissociation balance by alkalinizing the environment. This increases the duration of the anesthesia. The buffering capacity of the tear fluid (equals 8–10 microliter 0.01 N NaOH) is not sufficient to neutralize the instilled borax solution immediately. We therefore have under these conditions of the experiments with the same dose of local anesthetic more free alkali available. Our results correspond to those obtained by Soehring, Klingmüller and Neuwaldt (1959). Adriani and Zepernick (1964) found a slight increase in the duration of the anesthesia when Procain was instilled into an alkalinized tear fluid.

e) *The effect of various preservatives on the duration of anesthesia.* It is now mandatory that any bottle of eye drops which can be used repeatedly has to contain a preservative in order to protect the medication from contamination. It is, however, recommended to use these medications with preservatives only on uninjured eyes. Sterile one-dosage bottles are most desirable from a hygienic point of view and do not need any preservatives. They are especially suitable for the injured eye and for surgical interventions. In our experiments we were not interested in the antimicrobial effect of the preservatives, but only with the question whether they influenced the duration of the anesthesia. Our experiments showed that they do not have any side effect in this respect. It cannot be excluded, however, that in higher concentrations they could have such an effect. Klingmüller (1957) points out that they improve the wetting and penetration capabilities of surface anesthetics, but cautions against injurious side effects on the ocular surface. We may therefore postulate that the optimal effect of an ocular surface anesthetic depends not only the active agent, but also on the vehicle. These local anesthetic hydrochloride compounds represent an acid solution and their optimal stability lies in the acid range; the producers, therefore, have to attempt to dehydrate the solution and bring it as close as possible to the pH of a physiologic saline solution. Additives should only be incorporated when they are absolutely necessary, e.g. preservatives in bottles used for several applications (Brückner, 1973).

Macromolecules may interfere with the action of the preservatives (Klingmüller, 1957; Ophthalmica, 1975, page 141).

Additive surface-active compounds may also irritate. According to Lemp and Holly (1972), they may form a lipid emulsion and dissolve cell membranes. An improved absorption by the wetting action of the vehicle is usually associated with an irritation and therefore these compounds should not be added with the aim to improve the effect of the drug. An increase in the duration of the effect can be obtained by simply adding a few more drops of the drug (= increased dose).

Our experiences have shown that even the smallest amount (0.02 ml) from an eye dropper (i.e. one drop) of the usual surface anesthetic is sufficient to produce adequate anesthesia, e.g. to perform tonometry without that the patient shows any defense reactions. It is not recommended to prolong the duration of the anesthesia by increasing the concentration of the drug. It is noteworthy that the alkalinization of the precorneal film may by itself prolong the duration of the anesthesia because of a shift in the dissociation balance of the local anesthetic. It remains to be shown whether such a shift in the pH, e.g. by the application of a borax solution, would also have a beneficial effect on the anesthesia of inflamed tissues in which the pH lies on the acid side. The borax solution is unsuitable as a vehicle for local anesthetics because it accelerates the hydrolytic de-esterification.

# 15. Local Anesthetic Effects of Beta Blockers

Beta blockers have been frequently used during the last few years as a local glaucoma therapy. They lower the intraocular pressure by decreasing aqueous production.

Beta blockers have been used for 15 years in internal medicine for the treatment of hypertension, for cardiac arrhythmias and for coronary insufficiencies (Lands *et al.*, 1967).

The chemical structure of the beta blockers is quite similar to that of local anesthetics. This explains their membrane stabilizing effect (Morales-Aguilera, 1965).

Phillips *et al.* described in 1967 for the first time the ocular hypotensive effect of the systemically administered beta blocker Propranolol. This drug is poorly tolerated locally and therefore not suitable as a clinical treatment to decrease intraocular pressure (Vale, 1972).

Since 1974 we have in Timolol a locally well-tolerated beta blocker available which lowers intraocular pressure and is well soluble at a neutral pH value (Zimmerman, 1977; DeMailly, 1978; Nielsen, 1978; Bischoff, 1978; Krieglstein, 1978; Dausch, 1979).

Vale described in 1972 for the first time an undesired side effect of topically administered Propranolol and this occurs also after other beta blockers: a local anesthetic effect on the cornea.

This effect has so far not been quantitatively measured. Only Krieglstein (1977) investigated with the nylon thread esthesiometer of Cochet and Bonnet the local anesthetic effect of Bupranolol, another beta blocker.

We wanted to investigate this clinically important problem with the new electronic optical esthesiometer.

We also wanted to find out whether systemically administered beta blockers would affect corneal sensitivity as they also decrease intraocular pressure. This holds especially for Propranolol (Phillips, 1967; Pandolfi, 1974). This could be of decisive importance as the drug is extremely frequently used by internists.

## 15.1 Methodology

We compared various topically administered beta blockers (Draeger et al., 1980, 1982, 1983):

1. Propranolol in an 0.5% solution,
2. Bupranolol in an 0.5% oily solution,
3. Timolol in 0.25% and 0.50% and 1% solutions,
4. Metipranol in 0.25% and 1% solutions,
5. Pindolol in 1% solution.

We tested each medication on 20 subjects with normal eyes and on a corresponding control group. Their ages varied between 20 and 60. We limited the age range to 60 years as corneal sensitivity decreases beyond that age even without any medications (Boberg-Ans, 1956; Kemmetmüller, 1969).

We first determined the pretest threshold at 6:00 o'clock. We then administered one drop of the beta blocker into the conjunctival sac. We measured the corneal sensitivity at the same area every minute for 15 minutes. We established thresholds for the force necessary to elicit touch sensation. Measurements at the corneal center proved to be unsuitable as the normal threshold is here too low to be appreciably effected by the small local anesthetic effect of beta receptors.

When testing Bupranolol we had initially the impression that the local anesthetic effect could perhaps partly be due to the oily vehicle which changes surface tension. When testing the vehicle alone we did not find any local anesthetic effect.

We finally tested the local anesthetic effect of systemically administered Dociton = Propranolol on six patients. The dose varied between 80 to 120 mg/day. The average age of the patients was 50. We measured here the corneal sensitivity 1, 3 and 6 hours after the oral administration of the drug in order to appreciate also a possible late effect.

## 15.2 Results

1. Propranolol: Propranolol has by far the strongest local anesthetic effect. This effect appeared immediately just as in other ophthalmic local anesthetics. We divided the group of patients into a younger group between the ages of 20 and 40 and an older one between the ages of 40 and 60 as the two showed definite differences. The maximal threshold among the older age group rose to $320 \times 10^{-5}$ N. This higher value was maintained longer in the older patients than in the younger patients. The latter had the highest threshold of $300 \times 10^{-5}$ N (Fig. 53).

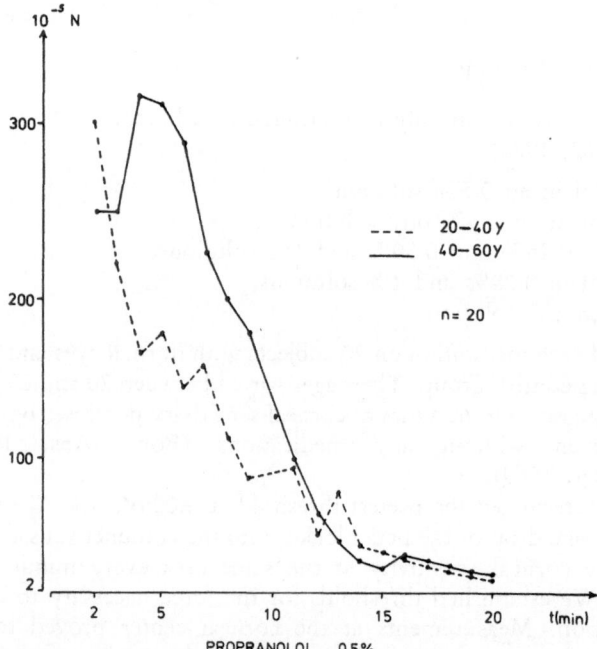

Fig. 53. Threshold after the application of 0.5% Propranolol

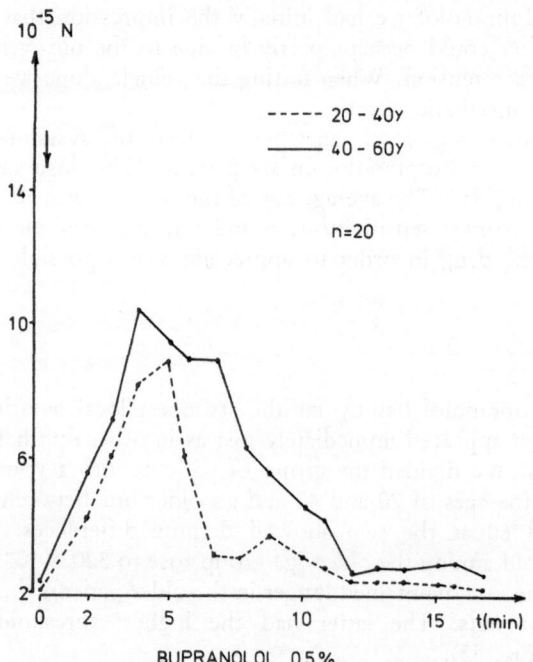

Fig. 54. Threshold after the application of 0.5% Bupranolol

2. Bupranolol: The local anesthetic effect occurred here also immediately. The maximal threshold among the younger patients was $8.8 \times 10^{-5}$ N and among the older patients $10.9 \times 10^{-5}$ N. This difference corresponds to the physiologic changes in corneal sensitivity with increasing age. After 15 minutes the pretest values were reestablished (Fig. 54).

The differences between the means is statistically significant with a p value of $< 0.001$.

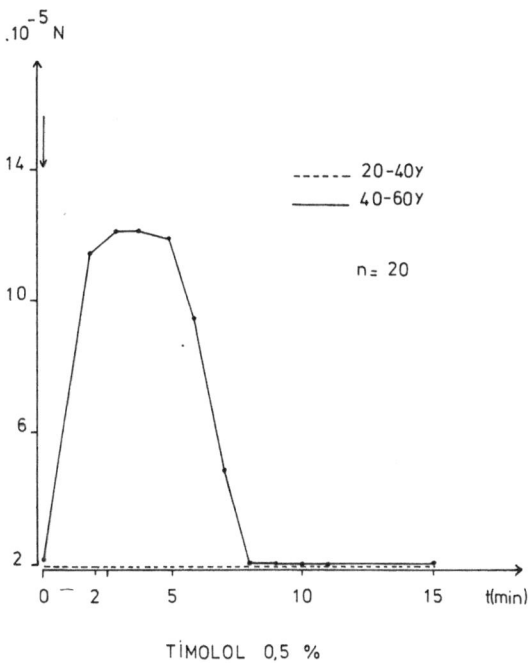

TIMOLOL  0,5 %

Fig. 55. Threshold after the application of 0.5% Timolol

3. Timolol: This drug had practically no local anesthetic effects upon the younger age group; among the older patients the effect reached immediately a maximal threshold of $13 \times 10^{-5}$ N. The threshold decreased rapidly after 6 minutes. The pretest values were reestablished after 11 minutes (Fig. 55).

4. We then tested Metipranolol in 0.25% and 1% solution. The results were practically the same as for Timolol (Fig. 56).

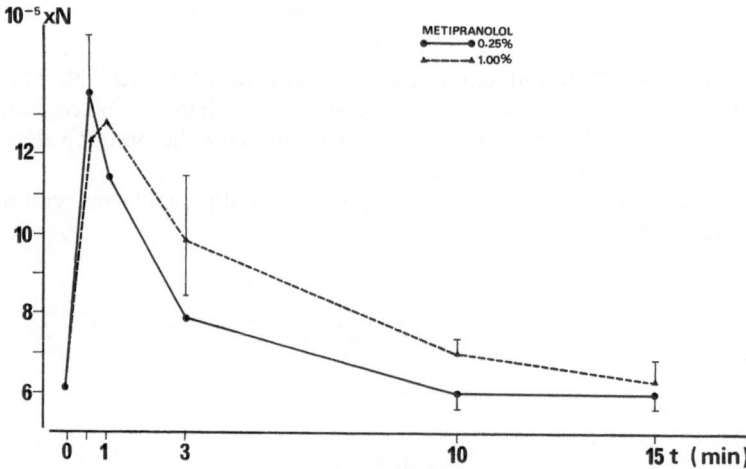

Fig. 56. Changes in corneal sensitivity after the application of 0.25% or 1%
Metipranolol

5. The results for Pindolol were the same as for Timolol and
   Metipranolol (Fig. 57).

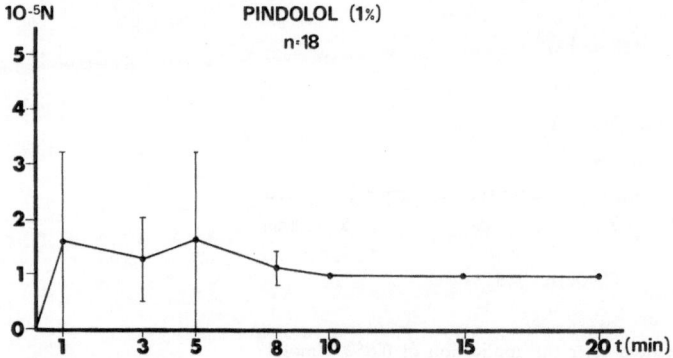

Fig. 57. Changes in corneal sensitivity after the application of 1% Pindolol

We subsequently tested a 0.25% against a 1% Metipranolol solution
and a 0.25% against a 0.50% Timolol solution in order to obtain a dose
response curve. The maximal effect is independent from the dose
applied. The recovery of corneal sensitivity is with higher doses
somewhat retarded (Fig. 58).

The oral administration of Dociton did not lead to any measureable
local anesthetic effect on the cornea.

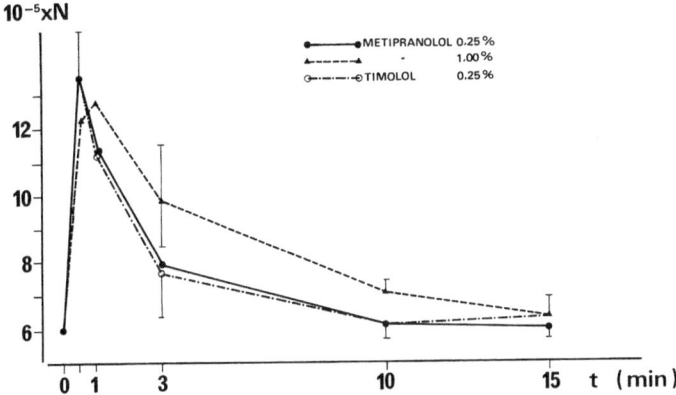

Fig. 58. Dose response curve of the threshold after the application of 0.25% and 1% Metipranolol and 0.25% Timolol

## 15.3 Discussion

It is well known that Propranolol and Bupranolol have a membrane stabilizing effect (Vale, 1972; Krieglstein, 1977; Stiegler, 1979). This could be confirmed by our measurements. In contrast to previous reports we found also for Timolol a local anesthetic effect, but only for patients between the ages of 40 and 60. The local anesthetic effect is small so that probably even after long-term use no damage need be feared.

We found no local anesthetic effect when beta blockers were given orally though, according to Krieglstein (1978), a dosage of only 60 mg/day corresponds to 200 times the amount of an ophthalmic local application. The corneal concentration of Oxyphenbutazon when given orally in a dose of 10 mg will correspond to only 1% of the tissue level reached after topical application (Stierlin, Tams, Wilhelmi, and Draeger, 1973). These results can only with reservation be applied to beta blockers, but they could explain the absence of a local anesthetic effect after systemic Dociton.

In four subjects we observed an unusual course. They showed after the administration of beta blockers a strong local anesthetic effect of long duration. As an example we illustrate the changes of corneal sensitivity in a 33 year-old man after the administration of three different beta blockers (Fig. 59).

It is possible that these persons have a genetically determined enzyme deviation. We know that such genetic differences in the metabolism of medications occur (Schloot, 1978). We know of

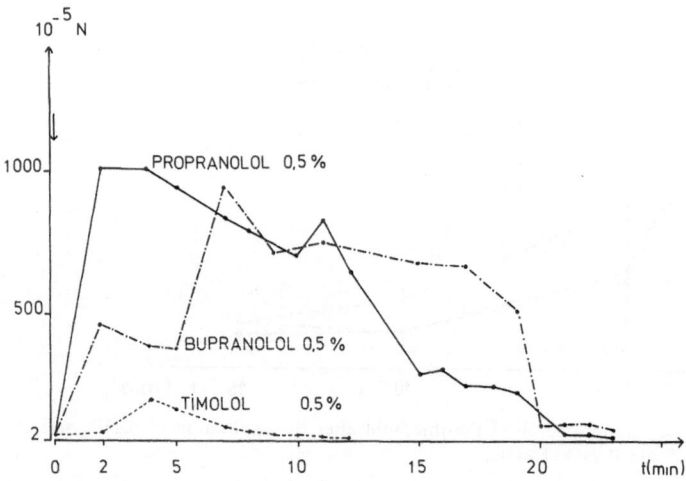

Fig. 59. Thresholds after the application of three beta blockers in one of the "responders"

genetically determined "responders," e. g. the taste sensation to Phenylthiourea. Armaly and Becker (1965) believe that the steroid response is due to a genetic variation. We made similar investigations in our clinic concerning the duration of the effect of Benoxinat. A similar, perhaps genetically determined, enzyme variation could be observed in the duration of the effect in 3 out of 15 subjects (see Chapter 16).

In conclusion, we believe that the local anesthetic side effect of the topically applied beta blockers does not in principle decrease their usefulness.

On the other hand, we have to keep in mind that in a few genetically marked patients these drugs may lead to a prolonged loss of corneal sensitivity.

We do not believe that there are any restrictions from an ophthalmologic point of view as far as the systemic administration of beta blockers is concerned.

# 16. Examinations on Pharmacogenetics

The individual genetic make-up of a patient usually determines the effectiveness and speed of breakdown of many medications; these are so-called pharmacogenetic reactions (Schloot et al., 1974 and 1976). In many of these cases of genetically determined enzyme defects or enzyme variations are normally latent. They become only manifest after the application of medications; in that way genetically determined syndromes can be elicited by the application of certain drugs.

These pharmacogenetically determined enzyme variants may manifest themselves in various ways:

– unexpected toxic side effects caused by the accumulation of the active agent = pharmacologic sensitivity or
– lack of therapeutic effectiveness because of precipitous degradation = pharmacologic resistance.

The enzyme may occur in several forms and when sampling a larger population a bi- or multimodal distribution may be found. Most of the pharmacogenetically determined protein or enzyme variants are extremely rare and occur as seldom as congenital metabolic disorders. Patients with the definite metabolic disorder lie outside the spectrum of the normal population.

Pharmacogenetic reactions on the eye have so far been only rarely examined and described.

Zistl et al. published in 1979 the first reports on variations in the speed of degradation for various surface anesthetics. They examined a sample of 31 subjects as to the effect of Benoxinat on corneal sensitivity.

The normal sensitivity for the corneal center was first determined for each individual; the center was chosen because it has the highest sensitivity. Four minutes after the application of the anesthetic, the corneal sensitivity was again measured with the handheld esthesiometer. These measurements were repeated every minute until normal sensitivity had been regained (Table 3).

Figs. 60 and 62 illustrate the correlation between the duration of the effect of Benoxinat in relation to the age of the subjects, for both sexes

Table 3. *Duration of the Effect of Benoxinat on Male and Female Subjects as well as on the Total Sample. Correlation of Regression Coefficients and Statistical Significance*

| Male Subjects (n = 15) | Female Subjects (n = 16) | Total Sample (n = 31) |
|---|---|---|
| $r = 0.482$ | $r = 0.458$ | $4 = 0.474$ |
| $p < 0.1$ | $p < 0.1$ | $p < 0.1$ |
| $b = 0.239$ | $b = 0.209$ | $b = 0.227$ |

r = coefficient of correlation; p = level of significance for the presence of a correlation; b = coefficient of regression.

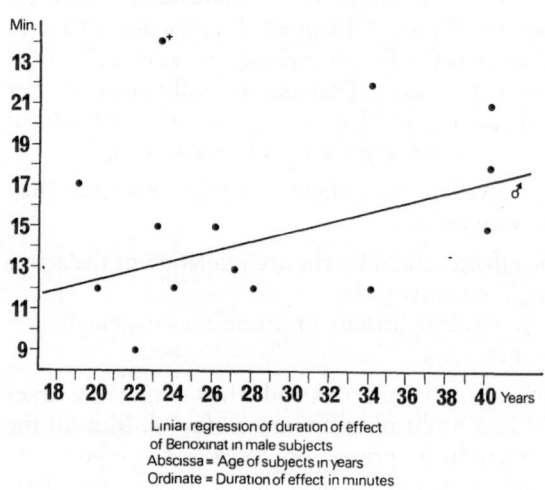

Liniar regression of duration of effect
of Benoxinat in male subjects
Abscissa = Age of subjects in years
Ordinate = Duration of effect in minutes

Fig. 60. Regression line for the duration of the Benoxinat effect among male subjects

and for the entire sample. Table 3 is a summary of the correlation and regression coefficients (Fig. 60).

By comparing the angle of the regression line for the entire sample, we find a regression coefficient which significantly deviates from the Null difference (b = 0.227); for the female subject this value lies at 0.209 and for the male subjects at 0.239 (Fig. 61).

In one male subject the value lies outside the range of all other male subjects, as well as outside the range for the entire sample. This therefore is a pathologic deviation with statistically significant differences. The subject and his family should be examined carefully to find out whether this is a familial trait and whether it follows a mendelian law. This extremely prolonged effect of the anesthetic could be due to pathologic changes in the transport of the drug or in a defective degradation of the medication (Fig. 62).

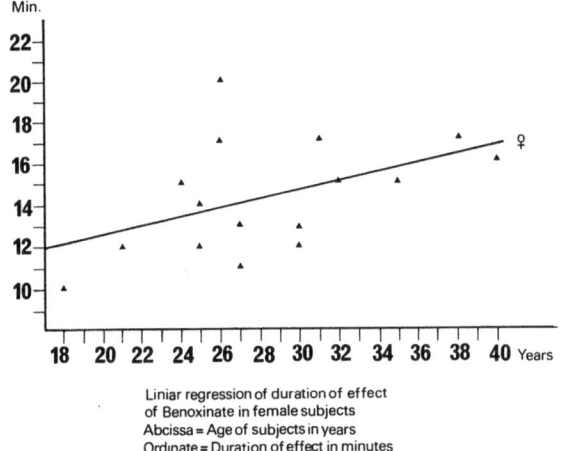

Fig. 61. Regression line of the Benoxinat effect for female subjects

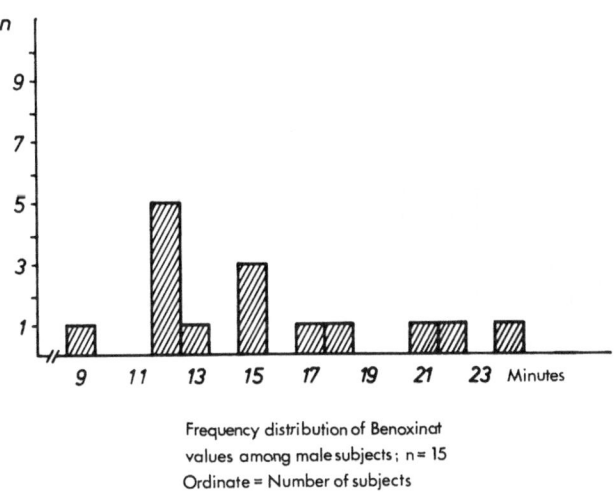

Fig. 62. Frequency distribution of the Benoxinat effect among male subjects; n = 15

The multifactorial analysis showed a significant increase of the Benoxinat effect with age; no correlation could be found with the sex, color of the eye, body weight or height of the subjects (Fig. 63).

We present in the Figs. 63 and 64 the frequency distribution of Benoxinat effect in order to determine whether we are dealing with a uni- or multimodal distribution. The values among the male subjects

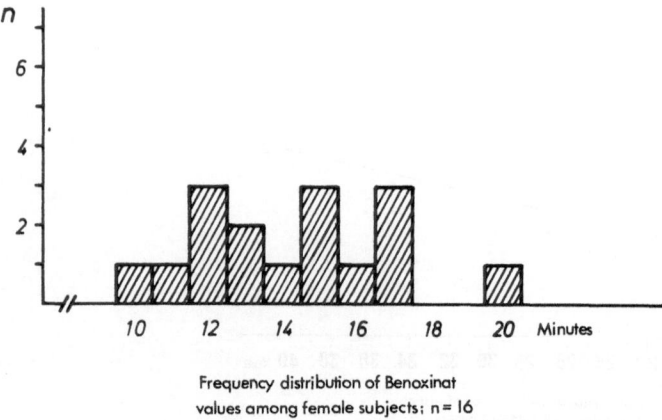

Frequency distribution of Benoxinat
values among female subjects; n = 16
Ordinate = Number of subjects
Abscisse = Duration of effect in minutes

Fig. 63. Frequency distribution of the Benoxinat effect among female subjects; n = 16

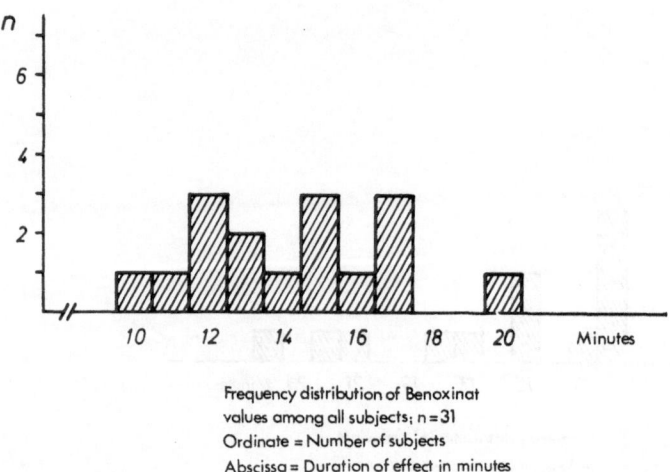

Frequency distribution of Benoxinat
values among all subjects; n = 31
Ordinate = Number of subjects
Abscissa = Duration of effect in minutes

Fig. 64. Frequency distribution of the Benoxinat effect in the entire sample; n = 31

show a considerable scatter (9–26 minutes); this is much less for the
female subjects (10–20 minutes). These two distribution curves, as well
as the one for the entire sample, did not allow us to come to any
conclusion whether this is a uni- or multimodal distribution pattern.
However, we can from these data not deduce that there is no
genetically determined polymorphism. We know of other examples
(acid erythrocyte phosphatase) in which an apparent unimodal

distribution encompasses several geno- or phenotypes (Edinger *et al.*, 1975) (Fig. 64).

We have to consider that even the normal corneal sensitivity depends in its various areas upon the age of the patient. There is a considerable decrease in corneal sensitivity beyond the age of 40, both for men and for women (Zistl *et al.*, 1979). It is noteworthy that among men beyond the age of 40, two groups can be differentiated which differ significantly in their corneal sensitivity.

# 17. The Influence of Contact Lenses on Corneal Sensitivity

It has been pointed out for years that wearing of contact lenses may change corneal sensitivity (Boberg-Ans, 1955; Hamano, 1960; Bryon and Weseley, 1961; Schirmer, 1963; Dixon, 1964; Kemmetmüller, 1969; Millodot, 1971, 1974, 1976, 1977; Larke and Hirji, 1979; Draeger, 1980).

The following reasons for this decrease in sensitivity have been mentioned: changes in the corneal metabolism, development of a corneal edema, changes in tear flow and creation of a relative hypoxia (Millodot, Kemmetmüller).

These phenomena are undoubtedly of great importance for the tolerance of contact lenses.

The questions therefore can be asked whether these changes in corneal sensitivity depend upon the mode of fitting, the material of the lens, the age of the patient, the refraction and especially on how long the contact lens has been worn.

It might also be interesting to investigate whether the corneal sensitivity of a prospective contact lens wearer would give us any clue as to his tolerance.

Numerous experiments have been made to answer some of these questions using previous methods to test corneal sensitivity (Kemmetmüller, 1969; Millodot, 1974, 1975, 1976; Schirmer, 1963).

At first we wanted to study retrospectively a series of patients who had worn contact lenses for some time and determine their sensitivity threshold. We selected 36 patients with polymethylmethacrylate (PMMA) and 37 patients with hydroxyethrylmethacrylate (HEMA) contact lenses. All of the patients had a myopia of moderate degree. All other eye findings were within normal limits, and especially the cornea was normal. Their ages varied between 23 and 35 years (Draeger et al., 1980).

We also initiated a prospective study which should show us in which way wearing of contact lenses could change the original corneal sensitivity. We selected 20 patients who then wore a hard PMMA contact lens and 15 patients who then wore a soft HEMA contact lens.

Their ocular status and age range corresponded exactly to the previous group.

The corneal sensitivity was measured before the contact lens was fitted, one week later, six weeks later and three hours after the contact lens had been removed.

We obtained all measurements, both for the retrospective and for the prospective study, in the vertical meridian, i. e. in the corneal center and at 6:00 o'clock at the limbus. All measurements were taken between 3:00 and 6:00 o'clock p. m. The patients had worn the contact lens on that day at least six to eight hours.

The PMM lenses had a diameter of 9 mm, the HEMA lenses a diameter of 13 mm.

# 17.1 Retrospective Study

## 17.1.1 PMMA Contact Lenses

For the first two years of wearing a contact lens the sensitivity threshold of the corneal center rises continuously and reaches a value

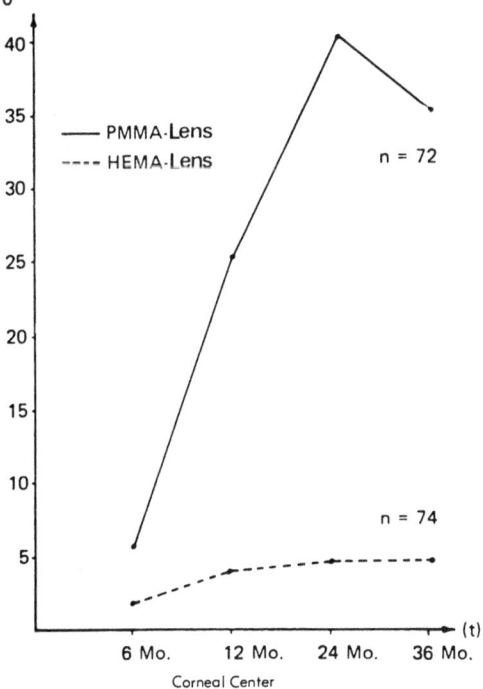

Fig. 65. Corneal sensitivity when wearing a PMMA or HEMA contact lens for three years; measurements at the corneal center

20 times higher than normal. After that time the corneal sensitivity apparently does not decrease anymore (Fig. 65).

The same results were obtained at the limbus at 6:00 o'clock; the threshold is higher to begin with and therefore the sensitivity decreases even further. The maximum values are obtained after two years of wearing time (Fig. 66).

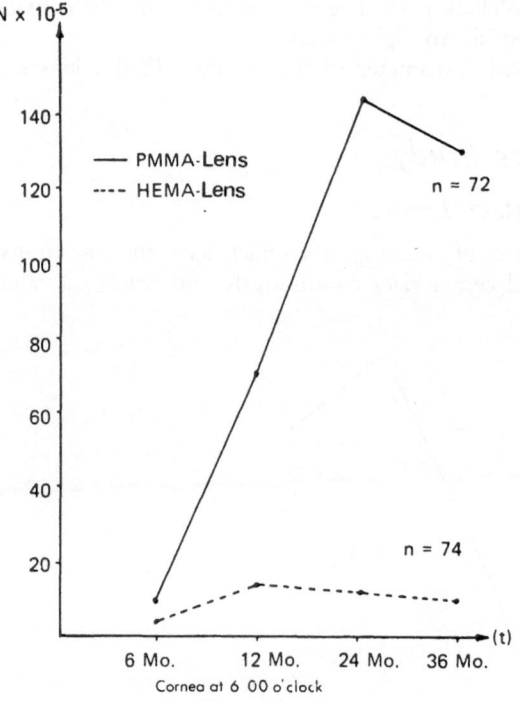

Fig. 66. Corneal sensitivity after wearing a PMMA or HEMA contact lens for three years; threshold at the 6:00 o'clock position of the limbus

## 17.1.2 HEMA Contact Lenses

We found a less pronounced, but still statistically significant increase of the threshold after wearing the HEMA lens. This applied both to the corneal center as well as to the 6:00 o'clock limbus (Figs. 65, 66).

The maximal decrease in sensitivity is here reached already after one year (Table 4).

Table 4. *Corneal Sensitivity at the Center and at the Limbus at 6:00 O'Clock After Wearing a PMMA or HEMA Contact Lens for Three Years*

| | | Center | | | 6:00 o'clock meridian | | | |
|---|---|---|---|---|---|---|---|---|
| | 6 mo. | 12 mo. | 24 mo. | 36 mo. | 6 mo. | 12 mo. | 24 mo. | 36 mo. |
| PMMA Lenses | Median = 5.7 | 25.5 | 40.36 | 35.4 | 10 | 70.4 | 143.4 | 130.7 |
| | Standard deviation = ±0.3 | ±6.4 | ±10 | ±8.5 | ±4.4 | ±36.3 | ±85.8 | ±55.3 |
| | Number = 16 | 16 | 24 | 16 | | | | |
| HEMA Lenses | Median = 2.0 | 4.5 | 5.0 | 5.0 | 5.0 | 15.5 | 14.5 | 13.2 |
| | Standard deviation = ±0.04 | ±1.3 | ±2.4 | ±2.8 | ±1.0 | ±2.0 | ±9.2 | ±9.3 |
| | Number = 22 | 19 | 18 | 15 | | | | |

# 17.2 Prospective Study

## 17.2.1 PMMA Contact Lenses

Wearers of PMMA contact lenses show an increase of corneal sensitivity in the center which after one week rises from $1.3 \times 10^{-5}$N to $3.5 \times 10^{-5}$N, i.e. by more than 100%! After another six weeks the corneal sensitivity decreased again somewhat. A corresponding behavior was observed at the limbus at 6:00 o'clock (Figs. 67, 68).

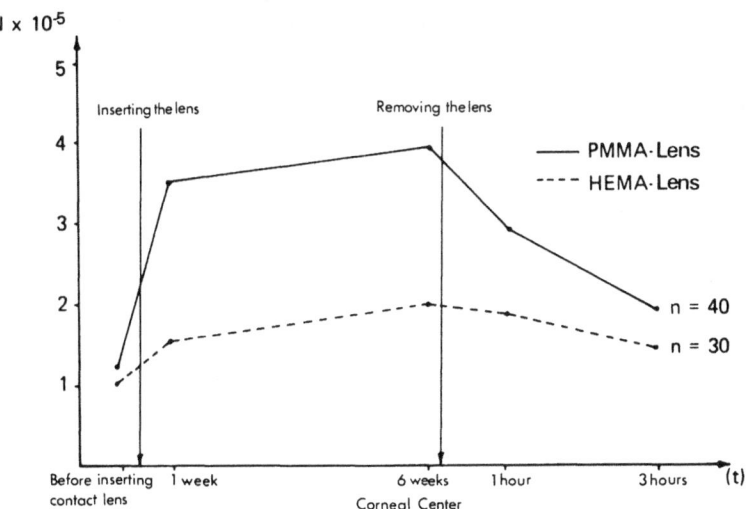

Fig. 67. Corneal sensitivity before and after wearing a contact lens. Comparison between PMMA and HEMA lenses, measurements at the corneal center

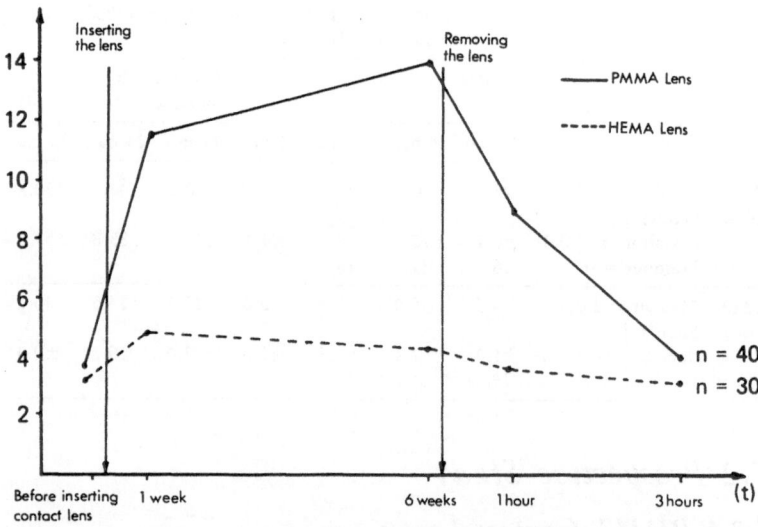

Fig. 68. Corneal sensitivity before and after wearing a contact lens. Comparison between PMMA and HEMA lenses. Measurements at the limbus at 6:00 o'clock

Most interesting was the behavior of corneal sensitivity after the contact lens has been removed: One hour after removing the contact lens the corneal sensitivity is already better than it had been after one week of wearing it. Three hours after removing the lens the sensitivity is nearly normal. This applies for the center as well as for the limbus (Table 5).

Table 5. *Corneal Sensitivity Before and After Wearing a PMMA Contact Lens, Corneal Center and Limbus at 6:00 O'Clock*

|  |  | PMMA Lenses | | After Removal | |
|---|---|---|---|---|---|
| n = 40 | Before fitting | After 1 week | After 6 weeks | 1 hour | 3 hours |
| Center | Mean value = 1.3 Standard deviation = ± 0.3 | MW = 3.5 S = ±1.5 | MW = 3.8 S = 1.8 | MW = 2.8 S = ±1.0 | MW = 1.8 S = ±0.3 |
| 6:00 merid- ian | Mean value = 3.5 Standard deviation = ± 1.0 | MW = 11.5 S = ±4.4 | MW = 14 S = ±3.8 | MW = 9 S = ±4.3 | MW = 4 S = ±1.3 |

In some of our patients we obtained values which deviated considerably from the mean. These were all wearers of the hard PMMA lenses and occurred in the center and at the limbus (Fig. 69).

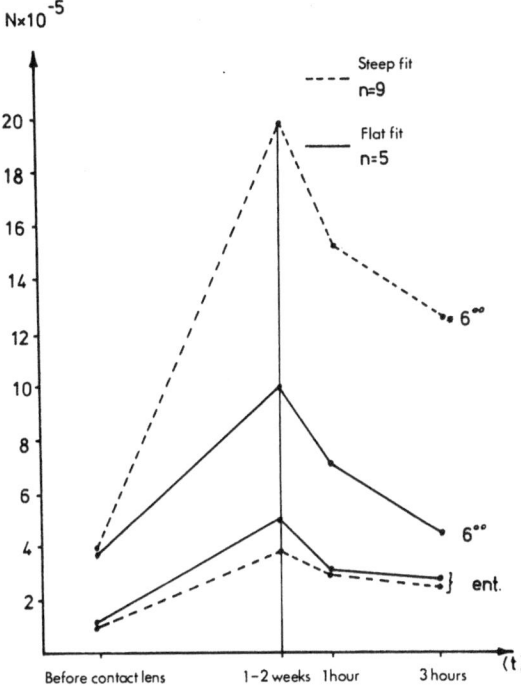

Fig. 69. The influence of fitting on the sensitivity topography of the cornea

An explanation of this unexpected finding was the definite correlation of corneal sensitivity to the type of fitting: Nine hard contact lenses which were originally fitted too flat, led to a more pronounced decrease at the center than at the limbus – i.e. just the opposite of the normal sensitivity distribution on the cornea! The condition was just the opposite in five contact lenses which were originally fitted too tight – the loss of sensitivity was more marked at the limbus (Tables 6 and 7).

Table 6. *Corneal Sensitivity When the PMMA Contact Lenses Are Fitted Too Flat*

|  |  | Flat fitting | After Removal |  |
| --- | --- | --- | --- | --- |
| n = 9 | Before fitting | After 1–2 weeks | 1 hour | 3 hours |
| Center | Mean value = 1.0 Standard deviation = ±0.2 | MW = 5.2 S = ±2.8 | MW = 3.2 S = ±0.8 | MW = 3.0 S = ±0.6 |
| 6:00 meridian | Mean value = 3.8 Standard deviation = ±0.09 | MW = 10.0 S = ±4.5 | MW = 6.3 S = ±2.5 | MW = 4.5 S = ±1.0 |

*Table 7. Corneal Sensitivity When the PMMA Contact Lenses Are Fitted Too Tight*

|  |  | Steep fitting | After Removal | |
|---|---|---|---|---|
| n = 5 | Before fitting | After 1–2 weeks | 1 hour | 3 hours |
| Center | Mean value = 1.0 Standard deviation = ±0.1 | MW = 3.7 S = ±0.9 | MW = 3.1 S = ±0.5 | MW = 2.5 S = ±0.6 |
| 6:00 meridian | Mean value = 3.8 Standard deviation = ±1.0 | MW = 19 S = ±7.2 | MW = 15.4 S = ±3.7 | MW = 12.5 S = ±5.8 |

The mechanical reasons for such findings are obvious if we consider the contact areas between the lens and the corneal epithelium in relation to the fitting (Fig. 70).

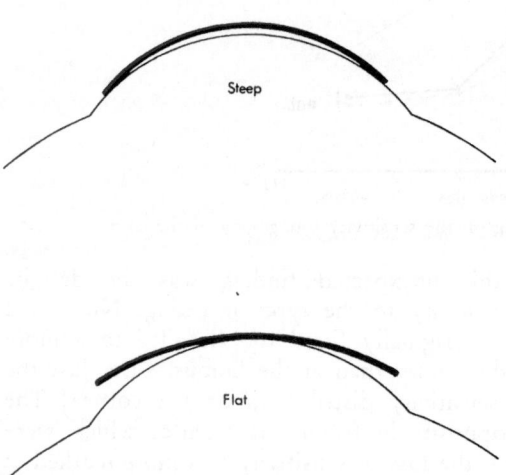

Fig. 70. Position of the contact lens, flat or tight fit

It took longer than the average in order to regain normal sensitivity when these hard lenses were removed. The increased contact between the lens and the epithelium has a longer lasting effect. We made the interesting observation that these patients had before a contact lens was fitted an unusually low sensitivity threshold. This corresponded to a relatively poor tolerance for these PMMA contact lenses. Patients who initially had a high sensitivity threshold showed usually later a better tolerance (Fig. 71, Table 8).

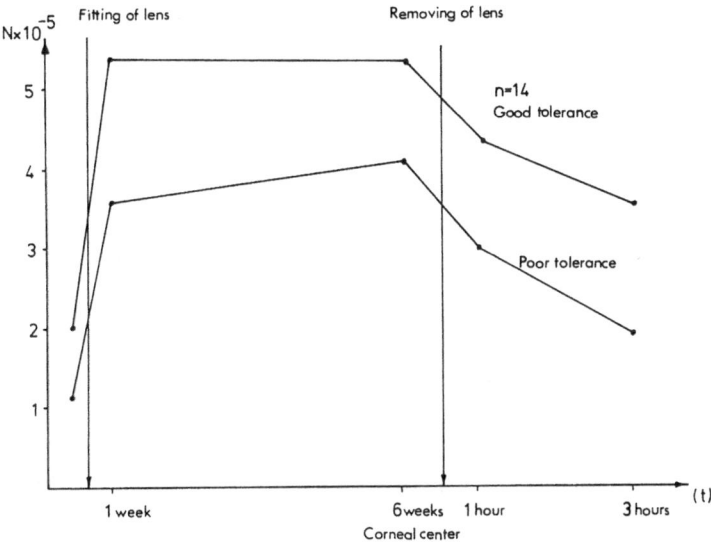

Fig. 71. Tolerance to PMMA contact lenses in relation to corneal sensitivity

Table 8. *Tolerance for PMMA Contact Lenses in Relation to the Sensitivity at the Corneal Center*

| n = 14 | Before fitting | PMMA Lens | | After Removal | |
| | | After 1 week | After 6 weeks | 1 hour | 3 hours |
|---|---|---|---|---|---|
| Center Poor tolerance | Mean value = 1.3 Standard deviation = 0.3 | MW = 3.5 S = ±1.5 | MW = 3.8 S = ±1.8 | MW = 2.8 S = ±1.0 | MW = 1.8 S = ±0.3 |
| Center Good tolerance | Mean value = 2.0 Standard deviation = ±0.09 | MW = 5.5 S = ±2.5 | MW = 5.4 S = ±2.6 | MW = 4.3 S = ±2.2 | MW = 3.5 S = ±1.3 |

## 17.2.2 HEMA Contact Lenses

We examined for this prospective study 30 eyes before and after fitting for HEMA lenses. We found here – similar to the retrospective study – only minimal changes in corneal sensitivity, both in the center and at the limbus. This occurred in spite of the fact that 6 contact lenses were originally fitted too tight and 4 too flat (Figs. 67, 68, Table 9).

The mode of fitting does in the case of the HEMA contact lenses not materially affect corneal sensitivity. There is not this type of contact with the epithelium as we see it with PMMA lenses. There is a

Table 9. *Corneal Sensitivity Before and After Fitting of HEMA Contact Lenses*

| n = 30 | | HEMA lens | | After removal | |
|---|---|---|---|---|---|
| | Before fitting | After 1 week | After 6 weeks | 1 hour | 3 hours |
| Center | Mean value = 1.0 | MW = 1.5 | MW = 2.0 | MW = 1.8 | MW = 1.5 |
| | Standard deviation = ±0.2 | S = ±0.3 | S = ±1.0 | S = ±0.1 | S = ±0.05 |
| 6:00 meridian | Mean value = 3.0 | MW = 4.8 | MW = 3.8 | MW = 3.5 | MW = 3.0 |
| | Standard deviation = ±0.2 | S = 1.0 | S = ±0.5 | S = ±0.8 | S = ±0.1 |

loose flat contact of the internal lens surface with the epithelium regardless of the type of fitting.

In conclusion, we can say that contact lens wearers, especially those wearing PMMA lenses, will experience considerable changes in corneal sensitivity; these changes increase up to a wearing time of two years. After that the corneal sensitivity reaches a plateau of a reduced sensitivity level. These changes are less pronounced in patients who wear HEMA lenses. This applies to sensitivity reductions in the center and at the limbus.

It is interesting to note that the type of sensitivity disturbance gives us a clue as to the mode of fitting: too tight a fitting influences more the limbus, too flat a fitting influences the corneal center. This rule does not apply to HEMA contact lenses.

These effects are not only due to a direct mechanical contact leading to pressure effects on the corneal epithelium and the anterior stroma; there is also a decreased oxygen supply as well as a thinning of the tear film. We also believe that the threshold of corneal sensitivity gives useful information as to the tolerance with which the contact lens may be worn. The ophthalmologist should regard any sudden drop of corneal sensitivity in a contact lens wearer as a potentially dangerous sign. It could point toward an increasing trophic damage to the cornea. Kemmetmüller has emphasized this in 1969.

It is well known that contact lenses can be well tolerated in an aphakic eye or after a keratoplasty. The reason is that these operations lead to long lasting sensitivity disturbances. We shall discuss this later on (see Chapter 18).

# 18. Corneal Sensitivity as an Indicator for the Reinnervation of the Cornea After a Cataract Incision or After a Perforating Keratoplasty

Corneal nerves are cut during certain surgical procedures on the anterior segment. This may lead to a partial or a complete loss of corneal sensitivity. The reinnervation can be studied on the basis of histologic examinations or clinically with the esthesiometer. Numerous authors have used one or both methods to investigate the recovery of corneal sensitivity (Cerise, 1908; Schröder, 1923; Marx, 1925; Babel and Campos, 1946; Franceschetti and Babel, 1947; Escapini, 1948; Kornblueth, Maumenee and Crowell, 1949; Maumenee and Kornblueth, Conner Moss 1949; Rexed, U., 1950; Rexed, B., and Rexed, U., 1951; Schirmer and Mellor, 1961; Kemmetmüller, 1969; Zorab, 1971; Ruben and Colebrook, 1979). These investigators used for the sensitivity measurements cotton threads, nylon threads, the hairs of v. Frey or the esthesiometer of Cochet and Bonnet. The determined time for the reinnervation varied greatly according to the method used. This is because with none of the previously available methods the threshold of corneal sensitivity can be determined exactly, nor can the extent of reinnervation be followed quantitatively. The cataract extraction and the perforating keratoplasty are classical models for such examinations – the corneal nerves are cut over a large area during the cataract incision and over the entire circumference during a keratoplasty. The donor cornea is after the operation completely anesthetic. Histologically, we find the following: The axon cylinder is 7 days after a keratoplasty slightly swollen; this swelling becomes more conspicuous after 12 days and after 30 days a large part of the axons is not recognizable anymore. After 60 days most of the nerves consist of empty tubes. These changes occur more rapidly in the host cornea than in the donor button. The nerves degenerate not only at the area of the incision, but up to 2 mm peripheral from it (Escapini, 1948; Kornblueth, Maumenee and Crowell, 1949; Rexed, U., 1950; Mensher, 1974).

New nerve fibers sprout from the trunks and grow toward the transplant. Many neurites can be seen after three to four weeks. They course toward the graft and originate from the trunks or from lateral branches (Rexed, U., 1950). At first they show a tortuous course toward the corneal center. Some of the nerves turn 90° as soon as they encounter the scar tissue and continue in a circular direction following the surgical scar. The irregular collagen fibrils of the scar present a considerable barrier for the delicate neurites. Once the scar has been penetrated the nerve fibers course again straight toward the corneal center (Escapini, 1948; Rexed, U., 1950; Zander and Weddell, 1955).

These new-formed neurites are first nude and not supported by schwannian elements. The schwannian cells of the graft do not degenerate. The neurites enter their empty sheaths and use them as directional tracts. In addition, there are also nude neurites without a sheath. After three to five weeks, a few neurites enter the scar; after three to seven months, we find a great number of mature nerve fibers in the graft. The first subepithelial neurites are seen after five weeks and after five to seven months the subepithelial nerve fibers net is complete. This growth pattern occurs whether the graft remains clear or becomes opaque. Occasionally the neural regeneration may be exuberant and irregular, so that a normal distribution and layering is not reestablished. The subepithelial nerves may be absent altogether (Babel and Campos, 1946).

If the graft becomes vascularized, nerve fibers will accompany the blood vessels. So far we may draw the following conclusions as to the reinnervation of the cornea after a keratoplasty. The following histologic stages can be distinguished:

1. The regeneration of corneal nerves is apparently independent from the transparency of the graft.
2. The reinnervation occurs from three sides:
a) The limbal end of the severed nerve bundle will send new axons toward the scar.
b) At the same time axons will proliferate circular around the scar and perforate it at a different point.
c) When not all fiber bundles are cut, e.g. after a cataract extraction, new neurites may sprout toward the scar. These come from below or from the corneal center and therefore innervate the surgical scar from the corneal side.

Schröder and U. Rexed believe that the last two possibilities predominate. Cerise, Escapini and Kornblueth, Maumenee and Crowell believe that the penetration of the scar by new-formed nerve fibers is more important.

## 18.1 Corneal Sensitivity After Cataract Extraction

We (Draeger and Martin, 1980) examined 227 patients between the ages of 26 and 90 after a cataract extraction with the handheld esthesiometer. The measurements were obtained at the corneal center, at 6:00 and 12:00 o'clock at the limbus, i.e. in the vertical meridian. In 99 patients the corneal sensitivity was tested before and after the operation. A retrospective group was checked up to eight years after the intervention. The prospective group had preoperative threshold values in the corneal center of $2.93 \times 10^{-5}$N, at 12.:00 o'clock $91.76 \times 10^{-5}$N and at 6:00 o'clock $33.60 \times 10^{-5}$N. The sensitivity at the limbus is in this group markedly lower than in a similar group of patients of equal age but without a cataract. We did not check whether a senile arcus with its typical local sensitivity decrease occurred more frequently among the cataract patients. The sensitivity values in the center corresponded to those of a similar age group of patients without cataracts. This result would speak for the assumption that the senile arcus could have been influencing our limbal values. It is of course possible that eyes with advanced cataract also have a high threshold of corneal sensitivity. The cataract may not only be an expression of a local disease process in the lens, but could be an indication for a metabolic disturbance of the entire anterior segment.

We tested the corneal sensitivity postoperatively after 7 days, 90 days, 1 year, 2 years and 8 years (Fig. 72).

During the first days after the operation, the upper corneal limbus and the center are practically anesthetic. When the corneal incision lies

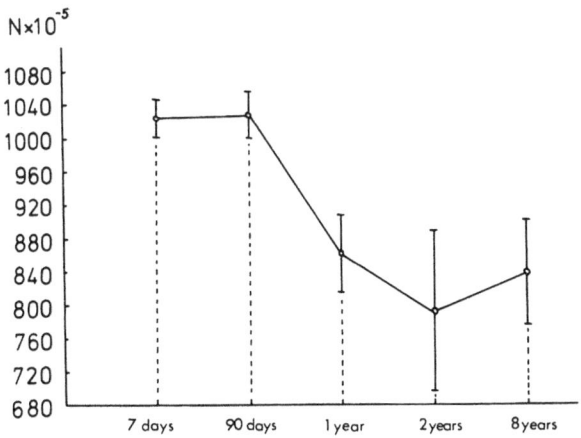

Fig. 72. Corneal sensitivity after cataract extraction, 7 days to 8 years postoperatively, 12:00 o'clock position at the limbus

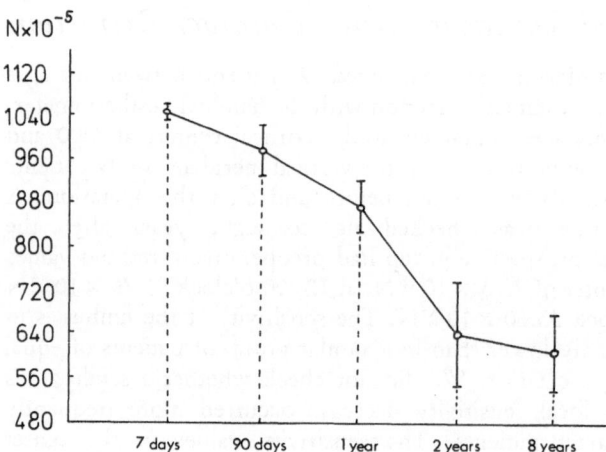

102    Corneal Sensitivity as an Indicator for the Reinnervation

Fig. 73. Corneal sensitivity after cataract extraction, 7 days to 8 years postoperatively, corneal center

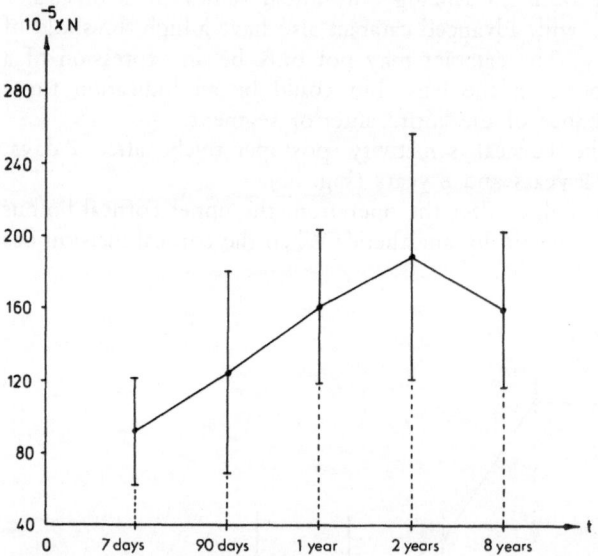

Fig. 74. Corneal sensitivity after cataract extraction, 7 days to 8 years postoperatively, the limbus at 6:00 o'clock

at the upper limbus nearly the entire upper half of the cornea will become intensive (Fig. 73).

These results contradict previous assumption that some nerve fibers could proliferate through three-fourths of the cornea (Zander and

Weddell). This should cause high postoperative thresholds for the corneal center. It is surprising that there is also a marked increase in the threshold at the lower limbus (Fig. 74).

There is a long lasting damage to the corneal nerves even in an area that is not affected by the incision. It is possible that there exists a long lasting trophic disturbance of the entire cornea involving also the area away from the incision. This would explain the increasing thresholds for two years after the operation; only after that time will the corneal sensitivity slowly return to normal values. Three months after the cataract extraction the corneal sensitivity at 12:00 o'clock is extremely low, practically nonexistent. During this time the scar represents a nearly unsurmountable barrier for the new neurites. The condition improves more quickly in the corneal center and this is probably due to a compensatory innervation of this area from the lower limbus.

Only toward the end of the first postoperative year will the reinnervation also be measurable below the surgical scar: the threshold improves now to $860.28 \times 10^{-5}$ N. The value in the corneal center is nearly the same, i.e. still markedly pathologic.

The best values are obtained at the end of the second year: $835.55 \times 10^{-5}$ N still present a considerably increased sensitivity threshold. There is no further improvement of corneal sensitivity during the following postoperative period. The slight increase of the threshold up to the eighth postoperative year probably represents only an age-dependent decrease of corneal sensitivity.

The value for the corneal center, on the other hand, improve during prolonged observation; however, they do not reach normal values (Fig. 73).

The following conclusions can be drawn from our investigations:

1. The upper margin of the cornea is practically anesthetic during the first three postoperative months. This improves gradually, but normal function is not reestablished.
2. The values at the corneal center are similar to those at the limbus during the early postoperative stage. Here also the sensitivity is practically extinguished. There is apparently no compensatory innervation from the lower limbus at that time. The recovery occurs later leading to lower thresholds than those at the area of the scar. Here too functional normalization is not achieved.
3. Surprisingly, the cataract extraction also leads to decreased corneal sensitivity at the lower limbus. This change is less marked than in the corneal center or in the area of the incision. Nevertheless, the decrease of sensitivity becomes more accentuated over a certain period of time.

Our results differ considerably from those obtained by previous authors. These differences are probably due to the more sensitive modern measurements. Previously, the corneal sensitivity was even in the healthy eye tested with suprathreshold values. This probably led to underestimating the loss of corneal sensitivity.

## 18.2 Corneal Sensitivity
### After Penetrating Keratoplasty

We examined 94 patients between the ages of 12 and 90 years. They had the following indications for the corneal transplant:

| | |
|---|---|
| Herpetic keratitis | 22 |
| Corneal dystrophies (e.g. Fuchs' dystrophy, keratoconus) | 28 |
| Bacterial infections, ulcer, old scars, injuries | 35 |
| Chemical injuries | 9 |
| Total | 94 |

Loss of corneal sensitivity is one of the main signs of a herpetic keratitis (see Chapter 16). Quantitative esthesiometry is not only important for a differential diagnosis of the herpes from other types of keratitis, but it also helps us in determining the course of the disease. It seems reasonable to assume that in such cases a penetrating keratoplasty will be accompanied by difficulties in reinnervation.

On the other hand, numerous authors have reported a quick recovery of corneal sensitivity after a keratoplasty for a Fuchs' dystrophy or a keratoconus (Escapini, 1948; Conner Moss, 1949; Müller et al., 1961; Günther, 1961).

In nonherpetic corneal ulcers the corneal sensitivity will be decreased only in the area of the ulcer or in its immediate surround. When the process is extensive the loss of sensitivity can involve also the accompanying edematous tissue (Boberg-Ans, 1955; Mensher, 1974).

The same applies to scars after perforating injuries (Boberg-Ans, 1955). In all of these cases we find a loss of corneal sensitivity which is less pronounced and more sharply delineated.

Chemical injuries, especially with alkalis, lead to the most severe trophic corneal damages. If the process reaches into the deeper stroma, the corneal nerves will be damaged; the sensitivity can be markedly affected. This impairs the possibility of reinnervation after a penetrating keratoplasty. Boberg-Ans, Mensher and Escapini have pointed this out previously.

We chose the following measurements for checking corneal sensitivity after a penetrating transplant: The sensitivity was measured on the transplant at 12:00, 3:00, 6:00 and 9:00 o'clock in a distance of 1 mm from the scar. Similar points were measured on the host cornea also 1 mm from the scar. The retrospective study extended up to eight years postoperatively (similar to the aphakic patients).

The measurements were obtained 6, 15, 36 and 100 months after the operation. As to be expected, the threshold was six months after the intervention $950 \times 10^{-5} N$, i.e. a practically anesthetic graft. The value is probably only a reflection of the mechanical transmission of the test object toward the adjacent parts of the host cornea (Fig. 75).

The threshold is even after 15 months exceedingly high. Only three years after the operation does the threshold begin to decrease and this

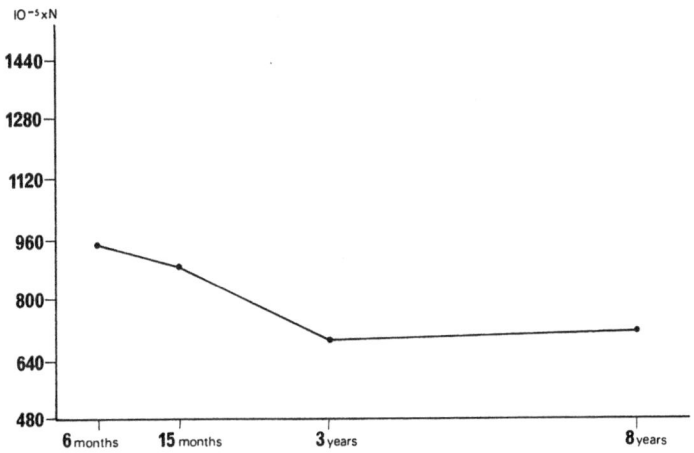

Fig. 75. Corneal sensitivity after penetrating keratoplasty, six months to eight years postoperatively, corneal center

Table 10. *Sensitivity Profile of the Cornea After Perforating Keratoplasty Obtained from Nine Different Points, Six Months to Eight Years Postoperatively*

|  |  | Up to 6 mos. | Up to 15 mos. | Up to 36 mos. | Up to 100 mos. |
|---|---|---|---|---|---|
| Center |  | 946.63 | 831.15 | 667.97 | 677.73 |
| Temporal | S | 671.54 | 232.59 | 300.10 | 308.33 |
| Temporal | W | 93.28 | 249.57 | 244.58 | 145.29 |
| Nasal | S | 613.43 | 300.20 | 380.85 | 374.44 |
| Nasal | W | 438.49 | 215.96 | 192.02 | 104.22 |
| Superior | S | 571.32 | 186.94 | 334.12 | 362.79 |
| Superior | W | 251.19 | 348.53 | 393.07 | 437.67 |
| Inferior | S | 491.93 | 154.17 | 307.40 | 251.29 |
| Inferior | W | 175.57 | 196.90 | 113.00 | 151.47 |

S = donor, W = host                                        $(\times 10^{-5} N)$

8    Draeger et al., Corneal Sensitivity

does not change materially during the further course of observation – the slight recurrence of an increase corresponds here also to the normal aging process.

Table 10 shows the thresholds for the topographic corneal profile during the entire period of observation (Table 10).

There is immediately after the operation a complete reversal of the sensitivity profile. In contrast to the normal profile the corneal periphery is now more sensitive than the corneal center (Fig. 76).

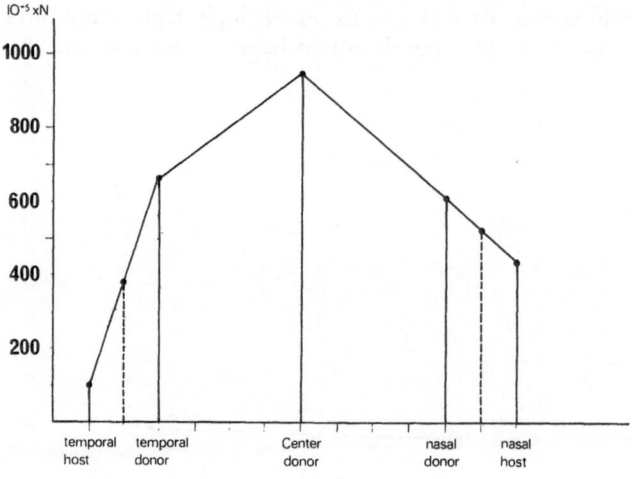

Fig. 76. Profile of corneal sensitivity after penetrating keratoplasty, measured in the horizontal meridian, six months postoperatively

As mentioned above, the center of the graft remains for a short time postoperatively completely anesthetic. The two values obtained close to the corneal incision probably represent only mechanical pressure transmission to the adjacent host cornea. We find in that area a much better, but still subnormal sensitivity – probably an expression of the retrograde degeneration of the cut nerves as we can observe it histologically. The vertical sensitivity profile is practically identical (Fig. 77).

There is a dramatic change after 15 months: The sprouting nerve fibers have apparently broken through the scar tissue (Fig. 78).

The threshold improves in the center, but is still subnormal. The same applies for the vertical profile (Fig. 79).

The measurement at the corneal periphery show that there is now again a tendency of the sensitivity to increase toward the center.

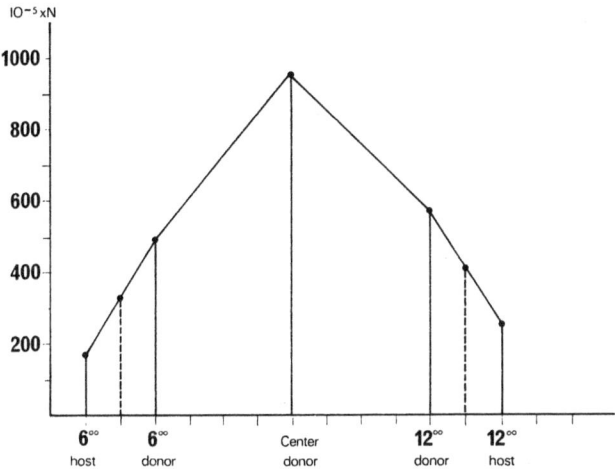

Fig. 77. Profile of corneal sensitivity after penetrating keratoplasty, vertical meridian, six months postoperatively

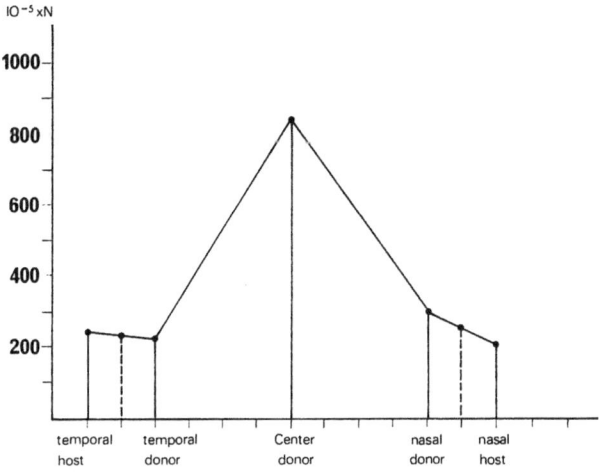

Fig. 78. Profils of corneal sensitivity after penetrating keratoplasty, horizontal meridian, 15 months postoperatively

However, the corneal center is not yet reached – probably because of the incomplete reinnervation in that area.

There is a further flattening of the sensitivity differential 36 months after the operation (Fig. 80).

8⁰

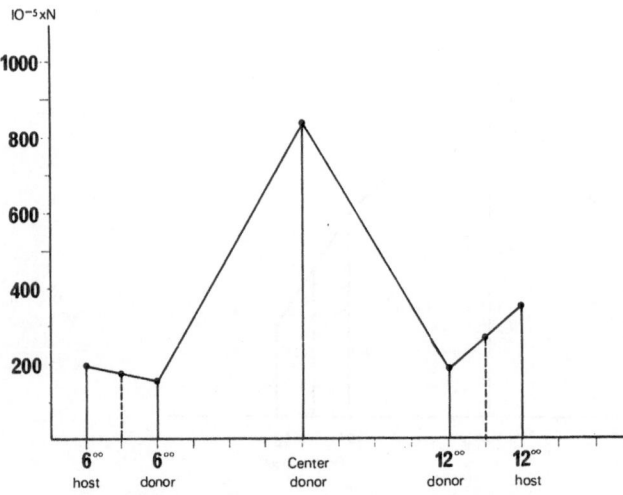

Fig. 79. Profile of corneal sensitivity after penetrating keratoplasty, vertical meridian, 15 months postoperatively

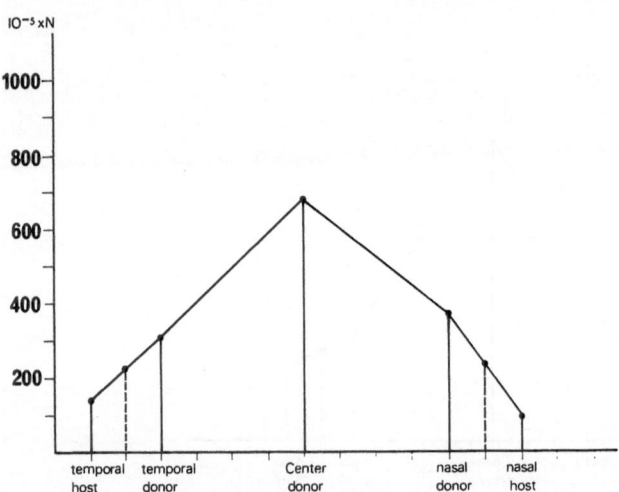

Fig. 80. Profile of corneal sensitivity after penetrating keratoplasty, horizontal meridian, 36 months postoperatively

The vertical meridian shows in the profile also a further flattening (Fig. 81).

Even eight years after the operation we still see the same reversal of sensitivity; there is no further improvement of the central sensitivity (Figs. 82, 83).

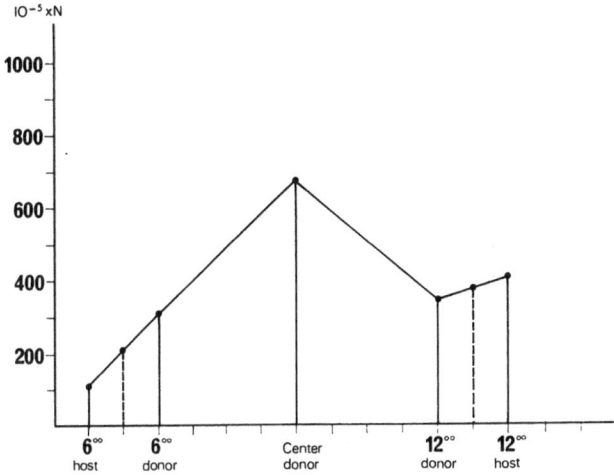

Fig. 81. Profile of corneal sensitivity after penetrating keratoplasty, vertical meridian, 36 months postoperatively

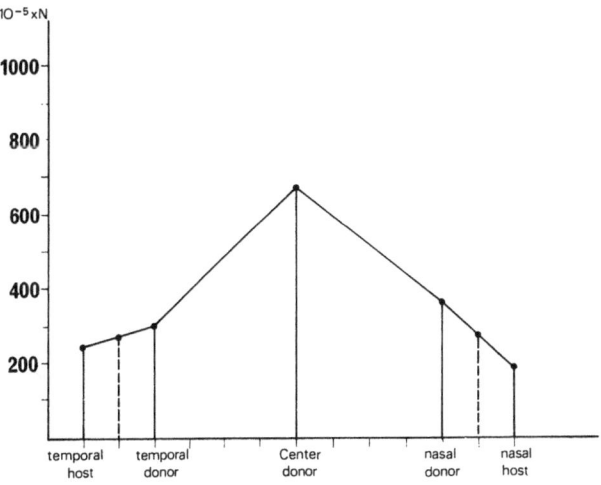

Fig. 82. Profile of corneal sensitivity after penetrating keratoplasty, horizontal meridian, eight years postoperatively

The mean values are somewhat misleading because when individual disease entities are evaluated separately the results are somewhat different: Some patients with corneal dystrophy show after two years again a completely normal corneal sensitivity or at least a normal profile pattern (Fig. 84).

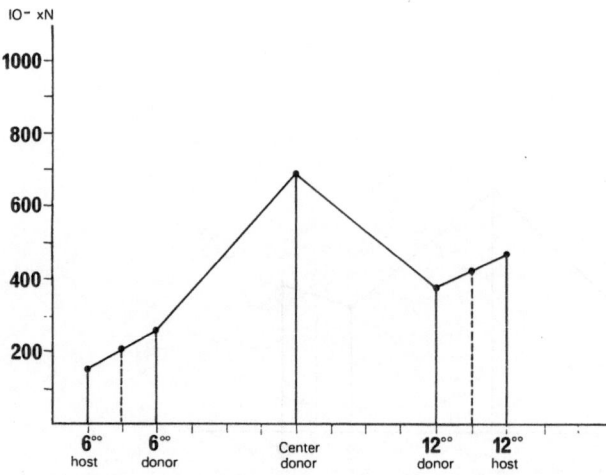

Fig. 83. Profile of corneal sensitivity after penetrating keratoplasty, vertical meridian, eight years postoperatively

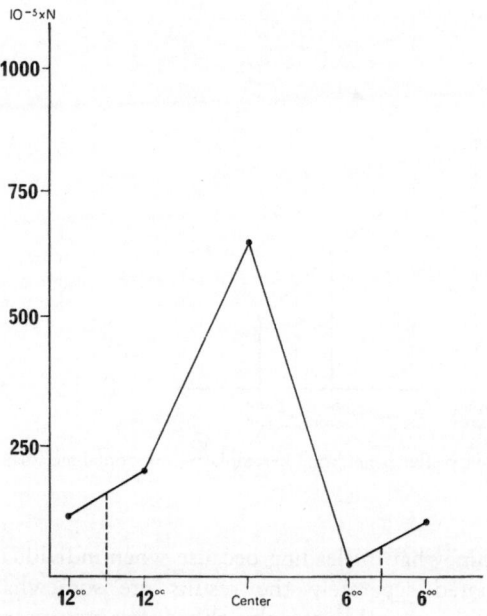

Fig. 84. Profile of corneal sensitivity after penetrating keratoplasty, two years postoperatively, corneal dystrophies

The discrepancy of the previously reported findings may be due to the fact that patients with different diseases were compared.

U. Rexed (1950) observed a recovery of corneal sensitivity after cutting the nerves; this occurred after four weeks when the experiment was done on young animals and after five to seven weeks when it was done on older animals. It took 7 or 13 weeks until normal values were reached (using much coarser examination methods). Escapini (1948) followed corneal sensitivity in albinotic rabbits for two weeks to nine months after the keratoplasty. He used cotton fibers as stimulus. The first reactions were obtained after 45 days in the corneal periphery. After 70 days the sensitivity had markedly improved. His experiments corresponded to his histologic examinations. The regeneration of axon cylinders somewhat preceded the recovery of sensory functions.

Kornblueth, Maumenee and Crowell (1949) also tested corneal sensitivity in the rabbit. They used v. Frey's hairs and obtained measurements between the 4th and 13th weeks. No individual reflex could be elicited up to the 6th postoperative week. Between the 11th and 13th week the corneal sensitivity for fine hair was reestablished. Conner Moss (1949) examined with v. Frey's hairs the corneal sensitivity after 24 penetrating and 2 lamellar keratoplasties. In 14 patients no reaction could be elicited even 10 years after the operation. On the other hand, 7 patients gave a positive response over the entire cornea and 4 patients responded only at a few measuring points. He found the first indications of the recovering sensitivity after barely 3 months. In one patient normal sensitivity was restored after 10 months. He did not find any correlation between the underlying corneal disease and the recovery of corneal sensitivity.

Ruben and Colebrook (1979) found in 48 patients with keratoconus a completely anesthetic graft up to one year after the operation. Some of the patients showed normal sensitivity values after three years, but in a few the threshold was high even six years after the intervention. Zorab (1979) performed follow-up examinations for two years after the operation. He found poor sensitivity in 44 patients, while 24 patients showed a better, though not normal threshold. Zorab also emphasized that there was no correlation between the transparency of the graft and the recovery of corneal sensitivity. Even completely anesthetic grafts may remain absolutely clear. Zorab, Ruben and Colebrook found a much lower corneal sensitivity than previous investigators had obtained on experimental animals.

This also applies to our results: Only 16 of the 94 eyes regained normal or nearly normal corneal sensitivity. The other patients had considerably higher thresholds and a few eyes showed a completely anesthetic graft even after a long postoperative period. We also found a direct relationship between the recovery time for corneal sensitivity and the age of the patient. A complete reinnervation occurred only in younger patients. Nevertheless, we have to assume that occasionally the corneal sensitivity may remain reduced after a corneal incision and the cornea will therefore remain vulnerable to touch and injury. The surgical trauma of a cataract extraction or a keratoplasty leads to considerable decrease in corneal sensitivity which affects corneal areas that are uninvolved by the incision itself.

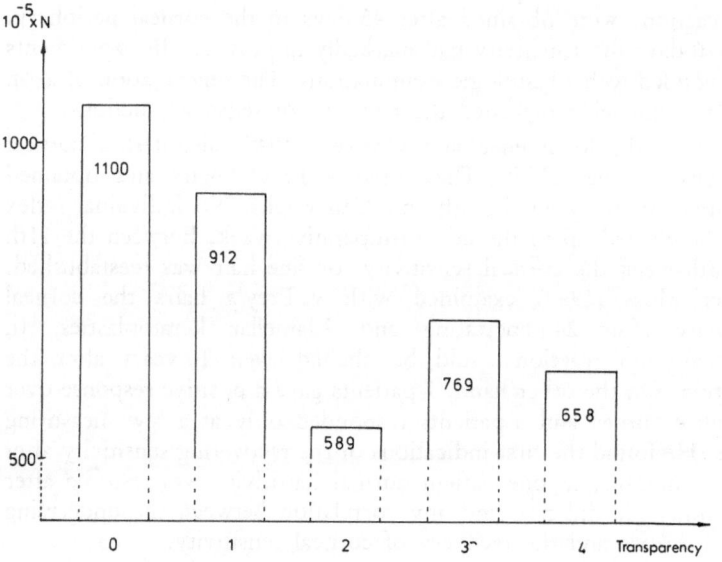

Fig. 85. Correlation between transparency of the graft and corneal sensitivity after penetrating keratoplasty

It has previously been attempted to correlate the transparency of the graft with the corneal sensitivity. The results of such investigations remained equivocal, probably because of methodological difficulties.

We also tried to correlate the transparency of the graft and evaluate it as an independent statistical parameter. However, it turned out that the postoperative visual acuity is a much better parameter, probably because it can be evaluated numerically while the definition of transparency is usually a subjective one.

The postoperative visual acuity can be correlated with the corneal sensitivity, both in the center and in the periphery. Increased sensitivity usually runs parallel with transparency (Fig. 85).

In eyes with cloudy grafts and therefore poor visual acuity – e.g. in the group of chemical injuries – we also find a low corneal sensitivity.

There is therefore a direct correlation between the trophic damage to the corneal tissues and the degree of reinnervation. It cannot yet be determined whether an anatomical and functional corneal reinnervation is a prerequisite or only an accompanying factor for the physiologic and metabolic normalization of the graft tissue. We believe, however, that measuring corneal sensitivity gives us an additional parameter – in addition to corneal transparency, corneal thickness and spectroscopic appearance of the endothelium – which allows us to evaluate the state of the graft. In addition, the corneal sensitivity can be measured at any time with accurate and reproducible results. It is quite likely that this will improve our prognostic capabilities as to the further course of a corneal graft in an individual patient. This may allow us to initiate the appropriate therapeutic measures at the correct time. There is an inverse relationship between the size of the graft and the speed of postoperative reinnervation, i.e. the larger the graft the longer the time required to restore normal sensitivity at the corneal center. This is due not only to the increased size of the scar barrier, but also to increased distance which the sprouting nerve fibers have to bridge. In addition, we have to keep in mind that eyes for which a large transplant was indicated are usually those that carry a poor prognosis. These eyes present a higher risk, show more often an opaque graft and a poor postoperative vision.

## 18.3 Comparison Between Fresh and Stored Donor Corneas

It is often difficult to get fresh donor material for a keratoplasty. It may happen that for a patient who needs an urgent or emergency corneal transplant the donor tissue is not immediately available. This may be due to the legal requirements in a specific country, to the poor cooperation with a department of pathology, or to the fact that appropriate donor material is must not available at that specific time. It has therefore been tried for a considerable period of time to store corneal tissue and to establish eye banks. It is possible to preserve corneal tissue for a long period of time by using rather sophisticated freezing and drying techniques. The operative results were satisfactory, though sometimes not quite as good as when fresh donor material was used. The logistics may be difficult, expenses and effort for such long-time storing procedures are considerable. In clinical practice it is usually not necessary to store corneal tissue indefinitely. It has only to be preserved until the next operation is scheduled. Much simpler methods are therefore quite satisfactory. McCarey and Kaufman (1974) have designed a practical way to preserve the corneas for a relatively short period of time. The corneal tissue can be kept alive when put into their media at 4° centigrade. Newer methods allow storage up to three weeks when using even higher incubation temperatures.

We had been using the McCarey-Kaufman method routinely for five years in order to store the corneas for a short period of time. However, this method was not used routinely and we were therefore in a position to compare the recovery of corneal sensitivity in eyes that had a stored cornea with those that had a fresh cornea for a corneal transplant (Fig. 86).

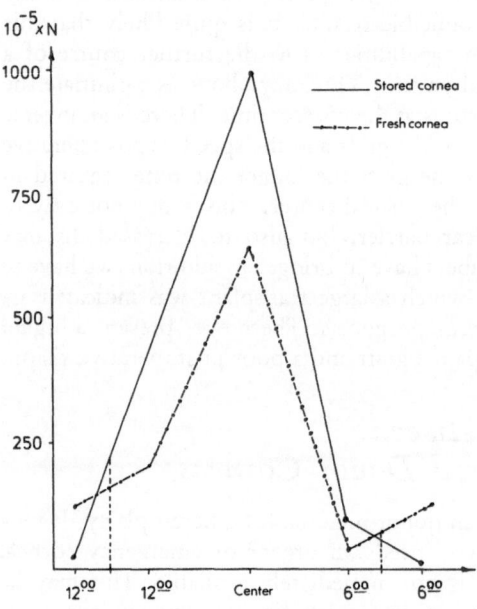

Fig. 86. Profile of corneal sensitivity in patients with Fuchs' dystrophy after penetrating keratoplasty, follow-up period: up to four years; age of patients: 40–60 years

The transplants performed with fresh tissue showed at any time a higher corneal sensitivity than grafts in which a stored cornea was used. The storage time varied between one to three days and the optimal time interval established by McCarey and Kaufman or by Bigar *et al.* (1975) was never exceeded. We therefore have to assume that there is apparently a certain trophic damage of the donor material when it is incubated in a nutrient solution and compared to fresh material.

Especially interesting is the situation in a 61 year-old man (Fig. 87).

This patient had a corneal edema and hyaloid touch after a cataract extraction. The other eye was blind because of a total retinal detachment. We therefore used the cornea of the blind eye as a donor.

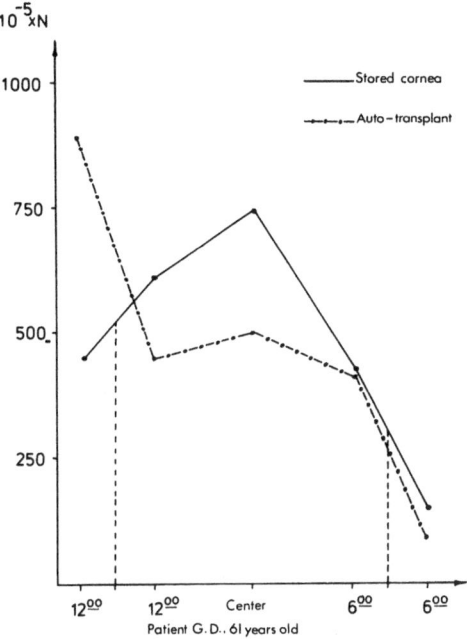

$10^{-5}$xN

Stored cornea

Auto-transplant

Fig. 87. Corneal sensitivity two years after a penetrating keratoplasty OD, 61 year-old man, auto-transplantation with the stored cornea from the other eye

A 7.5 mm graft was used and the defect in the blind left eye was replaced by a stored cornea which had been in an artificial medium for two days. The auto-transplantation occurred in one sitting without storage. The recovery of corneal sensitivity in the graft was extremely quick, while the threshold at the limbus of the host eye was still quite high. We may therefore assume that the relatively good corneal sensitivity of the graft is due to the excellent trophic condition of the donor material. The reinnervation began here from 6:00 o'clock in an area which consisted of relatively better stromal tissue.

On the other hand, the corneal sensitivity on the side where the preserved cornea was used recovered slowly. The values of the host corneal on that side were practically normal corresponding to the good condition of that cornea.

## 18.4 Reinnervation After Keratoplasty with HLA-Typed Donor Material

We thought it worthwhile to investigate whether the reinnervation of the corneal graft would depend upon the compatibility between host and donor tissues. The modern methods of storing corneal tissue (either for a long time by freezing and drying or for a short time by the modified McCarey-Kaufman method) makes it possible to perform tissue typing before the operation and to choose a donor tissue which is immunologically compatible. We therefore performed esthesiometric examinations after keratoplasties with donor tissue that had been stored for a short time. For one group of eyes the HLA compatibility had

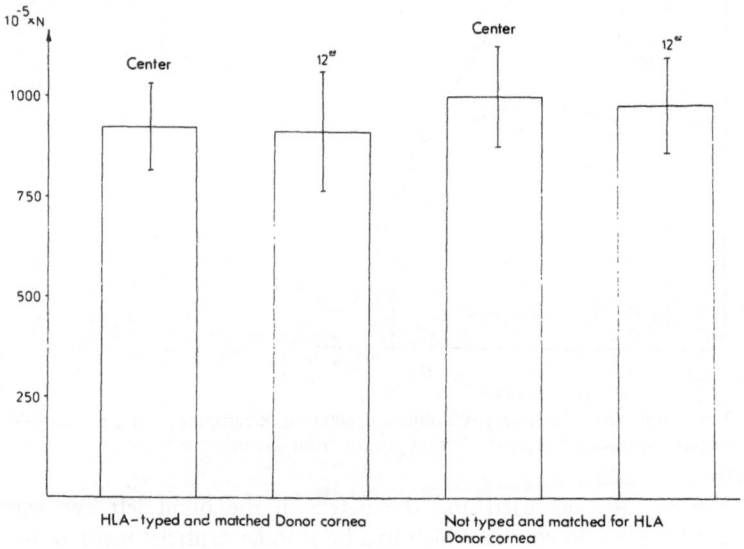

Fig. 88. Corneal sensitivity after keratoplasty, three months to seven years post-operatively, in relation to tissue typing

been taken into account. In the other group the operation was performed without that HLA tissue typing was considered. Differences in the recovery of corneal sensitivity were found in cases in which the keratoplasty was performed because of a herpes simplex infection of the cornea. These differences were obtained at the 12:00 o'clock position at the limbus and at the corneal center, though we find in every case of a keratoplasty after herpes a markedly decreased corneal sensitivity which, even after seven years, does not show a substantial recovery (see Chapter 18.2) (Fig. 88).

The results were different when the keratoplasty was performed for a corneal dystrophy. Corneal buttons which were grafted into an HLA compatible host did not show any better recovery of corneal sensitivity (Fig. 89).

A definite reinnervation could be found at the 12:00 o'clock meridian of the donor tissue three months to four years after the operation. The sensitivity increased to $384 \pm 554 \times 10^{-5}N$. Donor material which was not selected according to the HLA type and which was also stored for three days in a McCarey-Kaufman medium showed in the 12:00 o'clock meridian a sensitivity threshold of $693 \pm 479 \times$

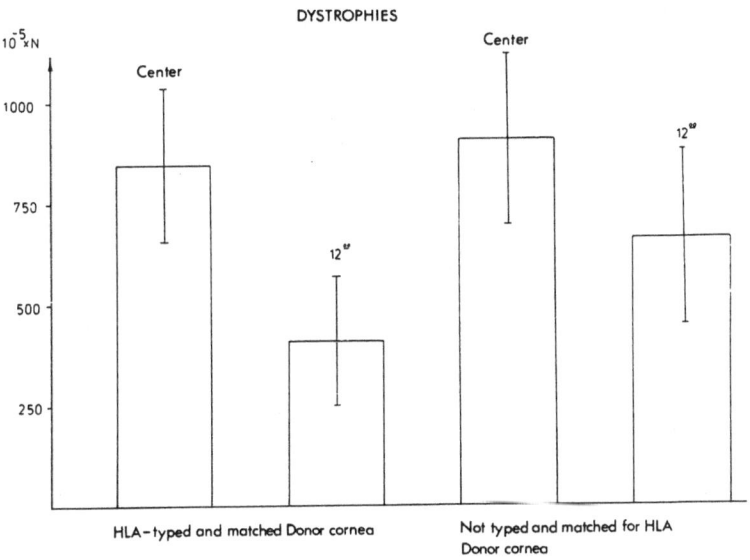

Fig. 89. Corneal sensitivity after keratoplasty for corneal dystrophies with HLA compatible or nontested donor material

$10^{-5}N$. No significant differences were found when the sensitivity was measured in the center of the graft. Both groups of grafts showed a markedly decreased sensitivity in that area.

In another series we determined corneal sensitivity in 42 eyes after a keratoplasty. The measurements were taken in the center of the graft, at the periphery of the graft and at 12:00 o'clock in the host cornea. All measurements revealed an extremely high threshold. We therefore could only differentiate two groups: one in which a threshold could still be measured and another one in which there was complete corneal anesthesia toward touch sensation. In the first group the patients perceived a touch sensation with the greatest amount of pressure; in the second group the patient did not indicate any sensation even if a force of $1100 \times 10^{-5}N$ was exerted.

The eyes could be divided into various groups according to the underlying pathologic changes which necessitated an operation:
The keratoplasty was performed for:

a) a herpes simplex infection of the cornea,
b) endothelial and epithelial corneal dystrophy (Fuchs' dystrophy),
c) keratoconus.

In 19 eyes the keratoplasty was performed because of a herpetic infection. No corneal sensitivity was found in three of these eyes in which the graft had been in place for only one year. A corneal sensitivity could be measured in 5 of the other 16 cases.

In 7 of these 16 eyes the graft had been matched after HLA-typing. To our surprise we found that in 4 of the 5 cases in which corneal sensitivity could be measured, the graft had been tissue typed and matched (Table 11).

Table 11. *Corneal Sensitivity After Keratoplasty for Herpetic Keratitis in Relationship to Tissue Typing and Matching*

| n = 19 | >1 year after keratoplasty | Matched for HLA | Not Matched HLA |
|---|---|---|---|
| Measurable corneal sensitivity (peripheral) | | $416 \pm 180 \times 10^{-5} \mathrm{N}$ | $600 \pm 250 \times 10^{-5} \mathrm{N}$ |
| Measurable corneal sensitivity (central) | | $825 \pm 220 \times 10^{-5} \mathrm{N}$ | $915 \pm 217 \times 10^{-5} \mathrm{N}$ |

The small number of cases does not allow any generalizations; nevertheless, we believe that there is a faster restitution of corneal sensitivity when the tissues of the donor and the host are matched than if they are used without HLA-typing. We have to consider, however, that in eyes with herpetic keratitis and subsequent keratoplasty the corneal sensitivity is severely reduced. There is already an anesthesia of the host tissue.

There was also no recovery of corneal sensitivity in the other group of patients one year after a keratoplasty for an endothelial-epithelial dystrophy. Nine patients could be observed for a longer period of time and there was no difference in corneal sensitivity whether the tissues were HLA-typed or not.

There is also no recovery of corneal sensitivity for at least one year after a keratoplasty performed for a keratoconus. Five patients could be observed for a longer period of time and there was again no difference in the recovery rate whether the tissues were HLA-typed or not.

Though the number of our cases in the various subgroups is still small, we are perhaps justified to draw some cautions conclusions. One year postoperatively corneal sensitivity is not yet reestablished. This has also been shown by other examiners. The recovery of corneal sensitivity among all groups of patients is not age-dependent. If corneal sensitivity recurs, it does so within two years after the operation and occurs first in the periphery of the graft and later in the corneal center. There was a correlation with HLA matching and restitution of corneal sensitivity only for those keratoplasties which had been performed because of a herpetic keratitis. In all other groups of patients such a relationship could not be established. This may be a spurious result due to the small number of our cases. On the other hand, it is wellknown that corneal transplants after endothelial dystrophy have, in general, a poorer prognosis than after a herpetic keratitis. The host has in these cases a generalized endothelial insufficiency which by the transplantation of normal endothelial cells will only be incompletely compensated. This also holds for secondary endothelial dystrophies, e.g. after a cataract extraction with vitreous prolapse or with severe endothelial trauma after an intraocular lens implant. Only when our results can be complemented by a larger number of patients can we make definite conclusions as to the influence of HLA-typing on the recovery of corneal sensitivity. Our first experiences seem to indicate that corneal sensitivity will recover more quickly and better if host and donor tissue have been matched for HLA characteristics.

# 19. The Influence of the Type of Anesthesia on Corneal Sensitivity

All local anesthetics used in ocular surgery will temporarily suppress corneal sensitivity. In principle, there are three different ways to initiate anesthesia:

1. surface anesthetics which are dropped into the eye and paralyze the receptors,
2. conduction blocks,
3. general anesthesia.

We have already alluded to the effect of local anesthetics on the receptors (see Chapter 9). This effect is dose dependent and can be prolonged by repeated instillations of the drug. There is normally no permanent damage of the sensitivity and the recovery is quick and complete.

The situation is less clearly defined in conduction anesthesia. We know that it is possible to produce long-lasting anesthesia if high doses are applied. This effect has been used for therapeutic purposes. The question therefore arises whether in addition to the previously mentioned local damage of corneal innervation (see Chapter 13) there could also be a permanent decrease of corneal sensitivity (Sedan, 1957).

We accepted as a working hypothesis that general anesthesia will not lead to permanent disturbances of corneal sensitivity.

We examined 207 patients after cataract extraction. Among them were 131 (63.3%) operated on under local anesthesia and 76 (36.7%) under general anesthesia.

Individual pilot measurements on patients after cataract extraction showed that after retrobulbar anesthesia corneal sensitivity was markedly decreased over the entire corneal surface. Snow and Sensel (1966) discussed the older, somewhat contradictory, results in the literature. They compared extensively the advantages and disadvantages of retrobulbar anesthesia in comparison with general anesthesia as far as modern cataract surgery is concerned. In evaluating the complications among 1000 unselected patients they found that, in general, local anesthesia was safer than general anesthesia. Some of then often cited disadvantages of general anesthesia can be avoided by modern methods, such as neurolepsy.

The present form of analgesia for neurolepsy with dehydro-benzperidol and fentanyl is especially suitable for the relaxation of a patient during the cataract extraction. Pöntinen, Miettinen and Rainikainen (1964 and 1966) have first emphasized this point. A disadvantage, however, is that the required dosage necessary for the introduction of anesthesia is difficult to calculate for an individual patient. The depth of the anesthesia may suddenly vary. This type of anesthesia also produces an annoying miosis.

During the anesthesia, whether it is general or local, the cornea will become completely unesthetic. The recovery of corneal sensitivity follows a definite course depending upon the site where it is measured. In the 12:00 o'clock meridian (Fig. 90).

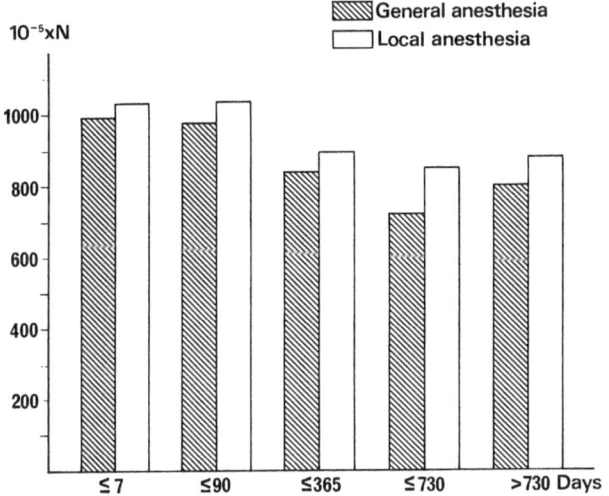

Fig. 90. Corneal sensitivity after a cataract extraction, measured in the 12:00 o'clock meridian, general or local anesthesia

This implies that close to the incision we find a nearly complete anesthesia for three months. After that the sensitivity returns slowly. Patients operated on under general anesthesia show a higher sensitivity. There is a decrease in corneal sensitivity two years after the operation for both groups of patients. This could be due to the advancing age of the patient group.

We find a similar recovery of corneal sensitivity in the center (Fig. 91).

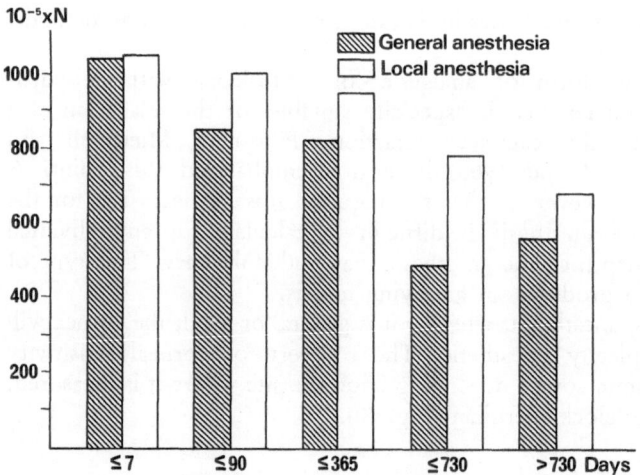

Fig. 91. Corneal sensitivity after a cataract extraction, measured in the center, after general or local anesthesia

Here also the postoperative recovery of sensitivity is better for patients after general than after local anesthesia.

We see a definite influence of local anesthesia in the 6:00 o'clock position, i.e. far removed from the corneal incision (Fig. 92).

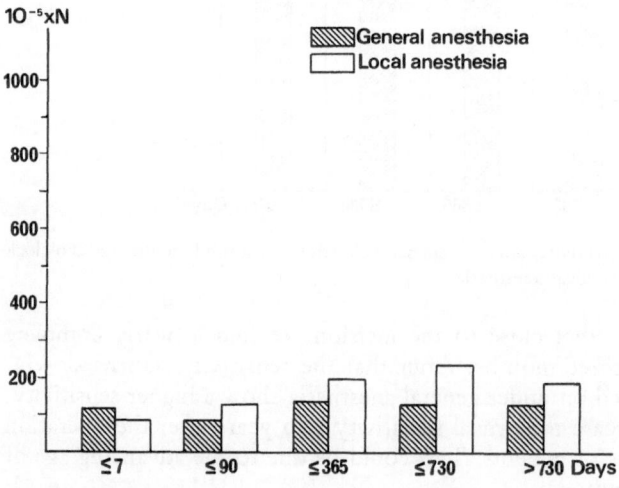

Fig. 92. Corneal sensitivity after a cataract extraction, measured in the 6:00 o'clock position, after general or local anesthesia

The corneal anesthesia is here after general anesthesia practically unchanged and resembles the preoperative values. We see practically normal values of corneal sensitivity for eyes operated on under local anesthesia also in the immediate postoperative period. The corneal sensitivity decreases, however, during the following two years and the threshold is higher than it was originally. This must be due to a long-lasting topical damage produced by the local anesthetic. After a long postoperative period (up to eight years) these differences between the two groups of anesthesia disappear again. The thresholds in the corneal center resemble each other and the values at the limbus do not change for patients who have been operated on under general anesthesia, while they improve slightly for patients operated on under local anesthesia.

We did not find any true damage of corneal sensitivity after a cataract operation performed under general anesthesia. The change in corneal sensitivity is in these patients due to the surgical trauma itself. After a local anesthesia the values for the 6:00 o'clock position remain normal in the immediate postoperative period, while corneal sensitivity decreases over the following two years. The threshold remains higher than the preoperative values or the values obtained on patients operated on under general anesthesia. The corneal sensitivity reaches nearly normal values two to eight years after the operation.

# 20. Corneal Sensitivity After a Buckling or Encircling Operation for a Retinal Detachment

It is not surprising that there is a damage to corneal sensitivity after surgical interventions on the anterior segment. In these cases there is usually a direct cutting of the sensory nerves. The situation is different after an operation for a retinal detachment in which changes in corneal sensitivity would not be anticipated.

So far there is little information available about the changes of corneal sensitivity after a retinal detachment operation (Ciurlo, 1965; Pannarale, 1965). Two factors of a detachment operation could influence the sensitivity:

1. a direct damage to the ciliary nerves as they course between the choroid and sclera. This effect is due to the surgically produced inflammation;
2. a damage of the ciliary nerves by compression due to the scleral buckle or a direct traumatic damage with a suture or by a surgical perforation.

In order to elucidate these problems we initiated an investigation of corneal sensitivity after retinal detachment operations.

We examined 35 eyes with a retinal detachment. In 15 eyes the corneal sensitivity could be studied prospectively and measurements were made before and after the retinal detachment operation. In 20 eyes the examinations were made only postoperatively. We used as comparison the fellow eye and measurements were made at the usual points, temporal, nasal, above, below and central in the cornea.

Among our patients were 28 women and 5 men; one of each group had both eyes operated on. These two patients could be measured preoperatively. The high number of female patients is a pure coincidence and is due to certain logistical aspects of the investigation. The patients were between 17 and 75 years old with an average of 59 years. Eight patients had a high myopia of more than −8.00 D; 9 patients had a moderate myopia and 4 eyes had an insignificant refractive error or were emmetropic.

We excluded all patients who had a systemic disease, e.g. diabetes or any other metabolic disorder, as well as patients who had another ocular operation either on the anterior or the posterior segment. There was an incipient cataract present in six eyes and this may have led to a somewhat higher effect of the coagulation treatment.

A silicone exoplant was applied to 42 patients (9 × parallel to the ora and 13 × radially); in 2 eyes the buckle was produced by an exoplant of dura mater tissue. A scleral pocket was prepared in 3 eyes, 5 eyes had a circumferential buckle and in 3 of these there was an additional vitrectomy with injection of gas into the vitreous space. For closing the tear a scleral diathermy was used in 5 eyes and in the other 30 a cryopexy was applied in order to close the hole. The corneal sensitivity was measured immediately before the operation, two weeks to six and a half years after the operation.

According to the surgical procedure we distinguish four groups of patient:

1. preparation of a scleral pocket with diathermy coagulation onto that area,
2. a silicone exoplant with cryopexy,
3. scleral buckle with cryopexy,
4. scleral buckle, vitrectomy and injection of gas into the vitreous space combined with cryopexy.

The results showed a surprising change in corneal sensitivity.

1. All five patients who had a diathermy application for the closure of the retinal tear showed considerable decrease in corneal sensitivity. In three of these patients the coagulation of a certain scleral area corresponded to a loss of sensitivity in the same corneal quadrant; in two patients in whom there was also a circumscribed area of scleral coagulation the loss of sensitivity extended over the entire cornea. This lasted up to six and a half years after the operation (Fig. 93). There was also a slight decrease of sensitivity in the corneal center when compared with normal subjects down to $2 \times 10^{-5}$N.

2. In 12 eyes the exoplant and cryopexy were applied only to one scleral quadrant. The postoperative decrease in corneal sensitivity was found only in the corresponding corneal quadrant. Because of extensive retinal changes the cryopexy had to be extended to two or several quadrants in another four eyes. The exoplant, however, was confined to one quadrant of the globe. The decreased corneal sensitivity was again limited to the corresponding corneal quadrants (Fig. 94).

In three additional cases there was loss of corneal sensitivity in all four corneal quadrants though the operation had been only

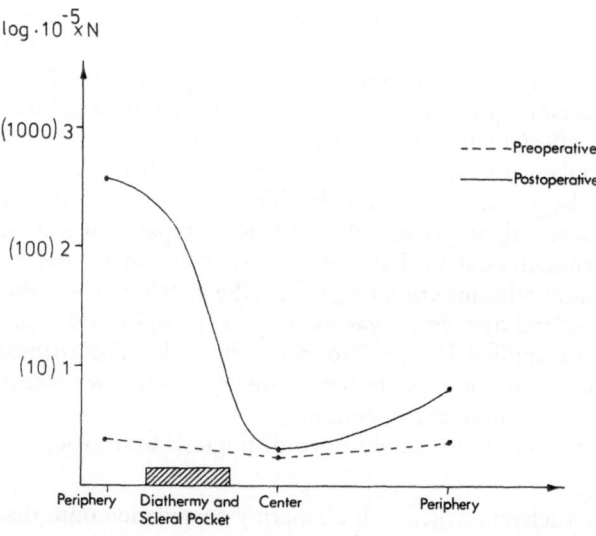

Fig. 93. Profile of corneal sensitivity in relationship to the scleral area treated and the corresponding corneal quandrant; group 1: scleral pocket and diathermy

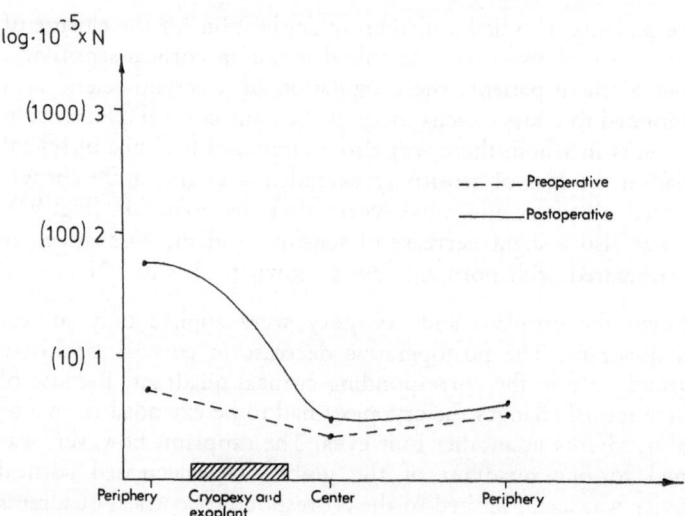

Fig. 94. Corneal sensitivity in relation to the surgical area; group 2: exoplant and cryopexy

performed over one scleral quadrant. These three eyes had before the operation a high bullous, nearly total or complete, retinal detachment. This required an extensive cryopexy during which large areas of the sclera were frozen. Central corneal sensitivity was also decreased. In three patients there was no change in corneal sensitivity over repeated postoperative examinations. The surgical technique did not differ from that in the other patients. The postoperative examinations were performed two weeks and one year after the intervention. These patients therefore did not experience any damage to the corneal nerves.

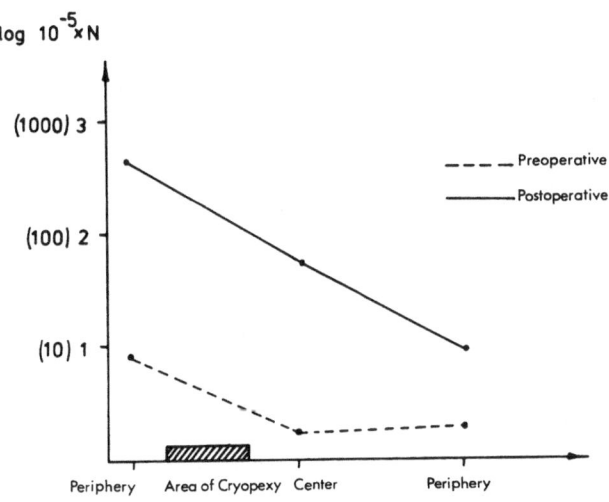

Fig. 95. Profile of corneal sensitivity in a 64 year-old man after scleral buckle and cryopexy combined with intensive light coagulation during the postoperative period

3. Five eyes had a scleral buckle because of multiple retinal holes. Cryopexy was performed in several quadrants and in these three eyes the corneal sensitivity was reduced in all four quadrants, though not to the same degree. One eye with high myopia and a macular hole was additionally treated by photocoagulation at the end of the operation and later on during the postoperative period. This eye showed a marked loss of central corneal sensitivity which could be due to thermal damage to the cornea during light coagulation (Fig. 95).
   Two patients did not show any change in corneal sensitivity.
4. In three eyes a vitrectomy with scleral buckle, circular cryopexy and injection of gas had to be performed (two of these patients had a

giant tear and one a massive preretinal proliferation). All three eyes showed a markedly reduced corneal sensitivity. The threshold were increased up to 400 to 1000 $\times 10^{-5}$ N (Fig. 96).

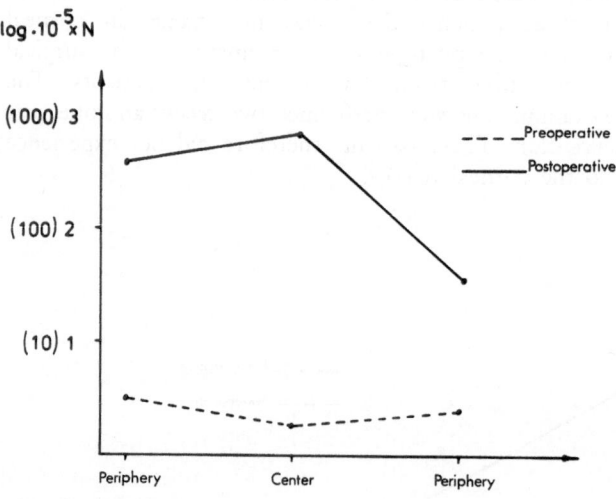

Fig. 96. Profile of corneal sensitivity after scleral buckle, vitrectomy, circular cryopexy and injection of gas

Postoperative measurements were only obtained up to one year after the intervention.

All of our examined cases showed after a detachment operation a marked decrease in corneal sensitivity. There is a certain relationship between the extent of the surgical intervention and the extent of the decreased sensitivity. In general, we find the reduced corneal sensitivity in the same quadrant in which the scleral procedure was performed. In cases of extensive cryopexy with long-lasting freezing of the sclera the entire cornea showed reduced sensitivity. This maneuver seems to damage the afferent nerve fibers which course close to the sclera. There is a partial interruption of their conductivity. Lyne (1977) described a reduced corneal sensitivity in patients with scleritis. This was reversible and the sensitivity became normal when the scleritis was cured. The same holds for changes in sensitivity after cryopexy or diathermy. The operation provoked not only a local retinochoroiditis, but also a scleritis. The diathermy has obviously a more potent inflammatory effect on the sclera and on the nerve fibers. Nevertheless, it is, because of the small number of patients, at present impossible to draw any definite conclusions as to whether the ciliary nerves are more damaged by diathermy coagulation. The duration of the coagulation, its extent and location determine the changes in an individual case and meaningful generalizations can at the present not be drawn. Nearly 85% of the patients with exoplant and cryopexy showed a decreased corneal sensitivity. In the majority of cases this affected only the corresponding corneal quadrant (or quadrants); in three eyes the entire cornea was affected. These three eyes had a bullous retinal detachment which required an extensive cryopexy which could have led to pathologic changes over a large scleral area. On the other hand, we observed three patients with identical surgical procedures who did not show any decrease in corneal sensitivity. In eyes with scleral buckle the corneal sensitivity was affected only in those corneal quadrants which correspond to the area of cryopexy. We found no instance in which the scleral buckle by itself due to mechanical pressure led to damage of the ciliary nerves.

Remarkable was the unusually pronounced loss of corneal sensitivity in three eyes which had been operated on with vitrectomy, cryopexy, scleral buckle and the injection of gas. Other cases with extensive cryopexy and scleral buckle showed only a minor loss of corneal sensitivity and therefore it is possible that the vitrectomy enhanced the effect of the cryopexy. In none of the eyes was the gas injected before the cryopexy. In such a case the cryopexy effect could be enhanced as gas is only a poor heat conductor. The vitreous may normally effectively dampen the effect of cold and heat.

Among 35 eyes which were operated for a retinal detachment, 30 showed a significant change of corneal sensitivity. We could not show any correlation between the time after the operation and the degree of sensitivity loss. Even five years after the invention there was considerable increase in the sensitivity threshold.

# 21. Corneal Sensitivity and Intraocular Pressure

It has been claimed for a considerable period of time that even a moderate increase in intraocular pressure can decrease corneal sensitivity (Luchik, 1966; Kalfa and Paramonov, 1955). They found in about half of the patients with increased intraocular pressure a decrease in corneal sensitivity. Awasthi and Goel (1969) confirmed the fact that corneal sensitivity decreases with age and with the height of the intraocular pressure. It is supposedly considerably decreased in angle closure glaucoma. Boberg-Ans (1955) showed that variations in intraocular pressure are accompanied by variations in corneal sensitivity. Millidot (1969) emphasized the connection between corneal thickness, corneal edema and decreased sensitivity.

Our investigations aimed to answer the following questions: Is there a correlation between intraocular pressure and corneal sensitivity? Is there a correlation between the duration of glaucoma and the threshold of corneal sensitivity and is it possible to draw from the corneal sensitivity any conclusions as to the cause of the glaucoma? It might be possible to use a corneal sensitivity measure for the diagnosis and prognosis of a glaucoma.

We measured the corneal sensitivity on 48 glaucoma patients (31 women and 17 men) between the ages of 30 and 79. We excluded patients older than 80 because of the unreliability of their answers and because of the rapid and marked decreased in corneal sensitivity at that age. We also excluded patients with any metabolic disease. All of our patients had primary open angle glaucoma.

As there is a correlation between the patient's age and the threshold for corneal sensitivity, we divided our patient material into two groups: Group 1 comprised patients between the age of 40 and 59 (17 eyes) and group 2 comprises patients between the age of 60 and 80 (70 eyes).

We measured the corneal sensitivity always at the same time of the day in order to avoid diurnal variations of the corneal sensitivity or of the intraocular pressure. We measured the sensitivity at the limbus at 6:00 o'clock. We also divided our sample into patients who showed a definite optic nerve damage and those who did not.

We found in our group 1 (age between 40 and 59) 17 eyes with normal optic nerves. These patients showed a threshold of $3 \times 10^{-5}$N. Unfortunately, there was in this group only one patient who had a definite optic nerve atrophy and he had a threshold of $8.5 \times 10^{-5}$N. A statistical analysis of this group is therefore impossible. Among the 39 eyes of group 2 (age 60–80) with normal optic nerve head the sensitivity threshold at 6:00 o'clock at the limbus was $4.40 \times 10^{-5}$N. Patients in the same age group with optic atrophy and glaucomatous excavation (33 eyes) had a sensitivity threshold at 6:00 o'clock at the limbus of $17.0 \times 10^{-5}$N.

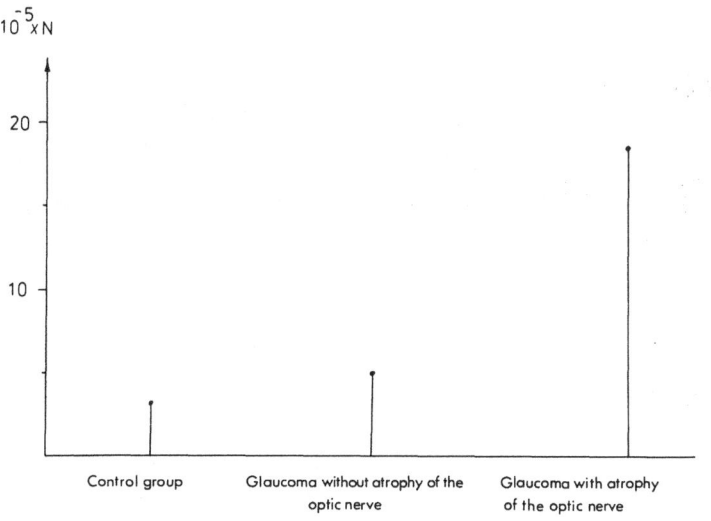

Fig. 97. The distribution of corneal sensitivity thresholds at 6:00 o'clock in normal and in glaucomatous eyes with or without normal optic atrophy

If we now compare the thresholds between patients with optic nerve damage to those with normal optic nerves, we find a definitely decreased threshold in the first group. If the glaucoma has already damaged the optic nerve, we also find damage to the corneal sensitivity.

The mean threshold for corneal sensitivity lies in patients of group 2 and with normal optic nerve quite close to the values of a normal control group. However, the distribution curves of the two populations is different. We find in the glaucoma eyes a second peak of high thresholds (Fig. 97).

We could not establish any correlation between the thresholds for corneal sensitivity and the duration of the glaucoma (Table 12).

Table 12. *Relation Between Corneal Sensitivity (Median Values) and Duration of Primary Open Angle Glaucoma*

| Duration of open angle glaucoma | Age group 1 (40–59 years) | Age group 2 60–80 years) |
|---|---|---|
| 1 to  3 years | 2 to 7 × $10^{-5}$N <br> Ø  3 × $10^{-5}$N | 2 to 69 × $10^{-5}$N <br> Ø   8 × $10^{-5}$N |
| 4 to 10 years | 2 to 5 × $10^{-5}$N <br> Ø 2.5 × $10^{-5}$N | 2 to 48 × $10^{-5}$N <br> Ø  4.5 × $10^{-5}$N |
| 10 to 15 years | – | 2 to 59 × $10^{-5}$N <br> Ø  4.5 × $10^{-5}$N |

We divided our glaucoma patients according to the median intraocular pressure in the affected eyes. We could not find any difference in corneal sensitivity among the patients with a median pressure below 20, between 21 and 25, or between 26 and 30 mm Hg (applanation tonometry) (Table 13).

Table 13. *Relation Between Intraocular Pressure and Corneal Sensitivity*

| Applanation tonometry | Group I (40–59 years) | Group II (60–80 years) |
|---|---|---|
| < 20 mm Hg | 3 ± 2.7 × $10^{-5}$N | 8 ±6.7 × $10^{-5}$N |
| 21–25 mm Hg | 3.2 ± 3.0 × $10^{-5}$N | 10 ± 5.8 × $10^{-5}$N |
| 26–30 mm Hg | 2.8 ± 2.5 × $10^{-5}$N | 11 ± 7.6 × $10^{-5}$N |

We found among our glaucoma patients a marked decrease of corneal sensitivity with advancing age. This exceeded the normal age related values and coincides with previous investigations (Luchik, 1966; Kalfa and Paramonov, 1955; Awasthi and Goel, 1969; Boberg-Ans, 1955). There is a remarkable difference in the threshold among glaucoma patients with or without optic atrophy. A long-lasting glaucoma which leads to excavation and atrophy of the optic nerve seems to damage also the sensory nerves of the cornea. We must assume that local metabolic changes caused by the increased intraocular pressure affect also the ciliary nerves.

We could not establish a direct relationship of corneal sensitivity with intraocular pressure or with the duration of the primary open angle glaucoma. A decreased corneal sensitivity is therefore not a reliable sign for the diagnosis of this type of glaucoma and cannot be used to make an early diagnosis. On the other hand, measuring corneal sensitivity might give us some clue as to the general damaging effect of the glaucoma, as a direct relation between a decreased sensitivity with optic atrophy could be established.

# 22. Differential Diagnosis and Monitoring of Herpetic Keratitis

Decreased corneal sensitivity played an important role in the diagnosis of herpetic keratitis even before Grüter (1930) could establish the etiology of this condition. Krückmann wrote in 1895 concerning corneal sensitivity: "The threshold is in this disease nearly always increased, not only in the area of the dendritic figure, but all over the cornea." "Decreased sensitivity of not affected corneal areas is pathognomonic for the superficial herpetic keratitis and is therefore of differential diagnostic value."

Pflimlin reported in 1930 various degrees of the disturbances of corneal sensitivity. He distinguished a febrile form of herpes, in which there was only a local decrease of corneal sensitivity in the affected area, from a constitutional herpes in which the entire cornea was involved.

Reiser (1940) could prove that there is in a herpetic keratitis nearly always complete anesthesia of the entire corneal surface. According to his investigations, this anesthesia lasts for months and, in deep severe herpetic infections, even for years.

Umbdenstock (1950) found a relation between the severity of the herpetic disease and the decreased corneal sensitivity. The more the sensitivity decreases the more severe will be the course of the disease. Measuring the sensitivity has therefore diagnostic and prognostic value. A markedly decreased sensitivity may also point toward frequent recurrences (Simkova, 1950).

An exact threshold determination was not possible with the older methods. We therefore re-examined a group of patients with herpetic keratitis and compared the results with a normal population. We determined the threshold profile in five positions (at the limbus at 3:00, 6:00, 9:00 and 12:00 o'clock and centrally in the cornea). After a keratoplasty we determined the threshold also in four additional points of the graft.

We classified the patients according to the severity of the clinical picture:

1. purely epithelial (dendritic) herpes,
2. recurrent epithelial herpes with beginning involvement of the stroma,
3. severe interstitial keratitis.

All eyes with herpetic keratitis showed a remarkable reversal of the normal topographic threshold profile (Fig. 98).

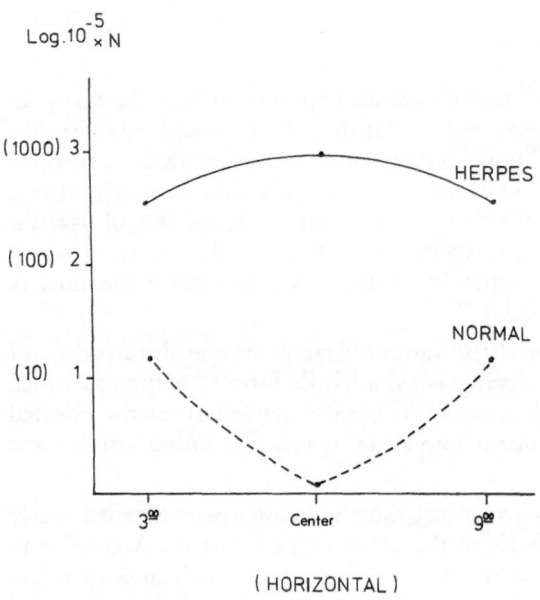

Fig. 98. Comparison of the threshold profile of normal and herpetic corneas

In the normal cornea the central area is the most sensitive part; in herpetic keratitis the highest threshold may be in the center. At the same time the threshold at the limbus will also increase, but not at the same rate as the corneal center (Fig. 99).

The center of the cornea is nearly anesthetic, in many of the eyes the limit of our instrument with a value of $1100 \times 10^{-5}N$ was reached. We therefore may regard this as complete anesthesia. There was usually some corneal sensitivity left in the periphery. The mean value of this sensitivity was around $400 \times 10^{-5}N$.

Other types of keratitis, e.g. a bacterial infection, will also show a certain decrease of corneal sensitivity. However, we never find this characteristic reversal of the sensitivity profile. We find in bacterial infections usually a more circumscribed focal area of decreased sensitivity which corresponds to the infected part of the cornea. The

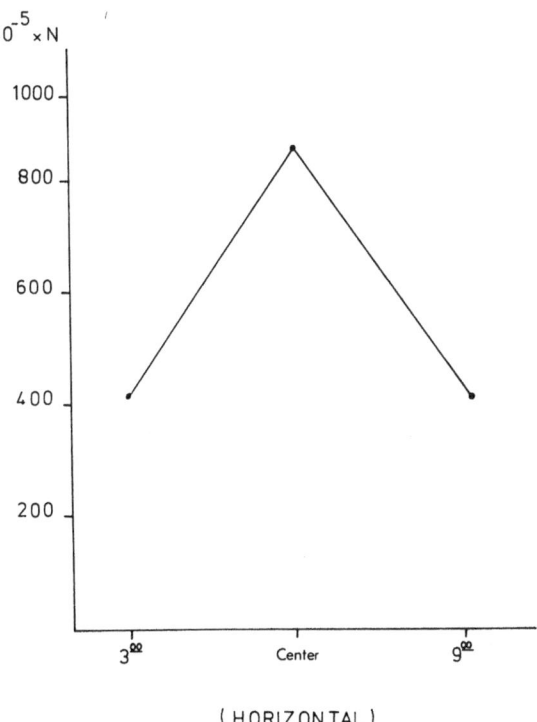

( HORIZONTAL )

Fig. 99. Topography of the threshold profile of all cases of herpetic keratitis

surround is in these nonherpetic infections usually completely normal and shows a normal sensitivity threshold. The degree of sensitivity loss corresponds to the severity of the clinical picture (Fig. 100).

The increase in the threshold is less marked in the dendritic type than in the interstitial form. We find in the superficial epithelial keratitis a central threshold of $250 \times 10^{-5}$N; in the recurrent keratitis the central threshold exceeds $800 \times 10^{-5}$N. In eyes with interstitial keratitis the cornea is often completely anesthetic at the center. There is still some sensitivity left in the periphery, but there the threshold is also markedly increased up to 500 or $600 \times 10^{-5}$N.

It is remarkable, however, that in some cases in which the clinical picture appears still rather innocuous the profile of sensitivity thresholds corresponds to the more severe infections: in these cases we are always dealing with a disease that had repeatedly recurred so that the damage to the corneal nerves was more severe than could be anticipated on slit lamp examination. Measuring the corneal sensitivity is therefore in these cases of prognostic value.

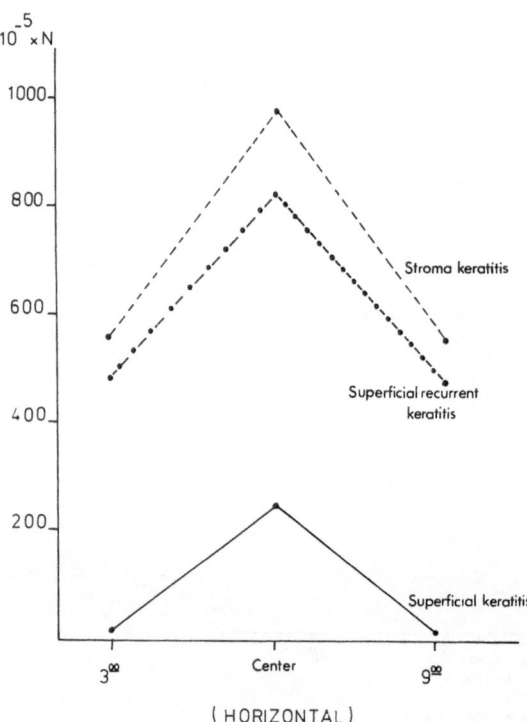

Fig. 100. Profile of corneal sensitivity in herpetic keratitis (epithelial, recurrent epithelial and severe interstitial types)

The severity of the disease also determined the duration of decreased corneal sensitivity. When the epithelial defect heals normal sensitivity will be reestablished. This occurs first in the periphery and then in the center (Fig. 101).

Even for the superficial keratitis the normalization of corneal sensitivity takes over two years. Recurrent superficial keratitis cases will also show considerable improvement of their corneal sensitivity provided no new recurrence has occurred. However, even after two years this sensitivity will not reach a normal threshold, at least centrally. In eyes with interstitial keratitis there is practically no recovery of corneal sensitivity.

The topographic threshold profile shows a similar course. A reversal to the normal profile takes up to two years in eyes with superficial keratitis.

Eyes with a herpetic keratitis of group 2 (recurrent epithelial lesions with involvement of the superficial stroma) show an improvement of

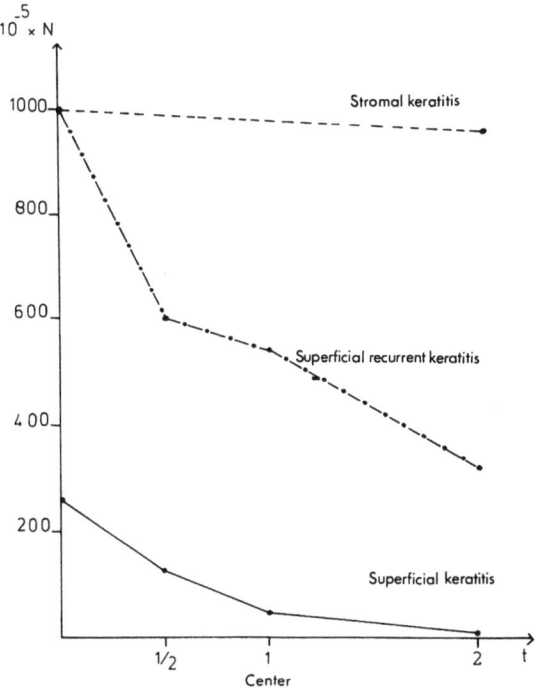

Fig. 101. Temporal course of decreased corneal sensitivity in herpetic infections in relationship to the severity of the disease (epithelial, recurrent epithelial and severe interstitial keratitis)

corneal sensitivity, but the typical reversal remains for a long time or permanently, i. e. there remains a central hyposensitivity. In one woman we found over three years a complete anesthesia of the corneal center though clinically the cornea had healed with the formation of scars and there was certainly no recurrence.

The profile of corneal sensitivity after a keratoplasty for a herpetic keratitis has to be compared with the corneal sensitivity when the keratoplasty was performed for a nonherpetic corneal affection (Fig. 102).

We normally find immediately postoperatively a central anesthesia because the corneal nerves have been cut. Reinnervation occurs only two to three years later when the nerves sprout into the graft. Seven years after the operation the threshold is in the corneal center again lower than in the corneal periphery, i. e. the typical topographic profile of corneal sensitivity has been reestablished, though the values are higher than normal. The course is entirely different after a keratoplasty

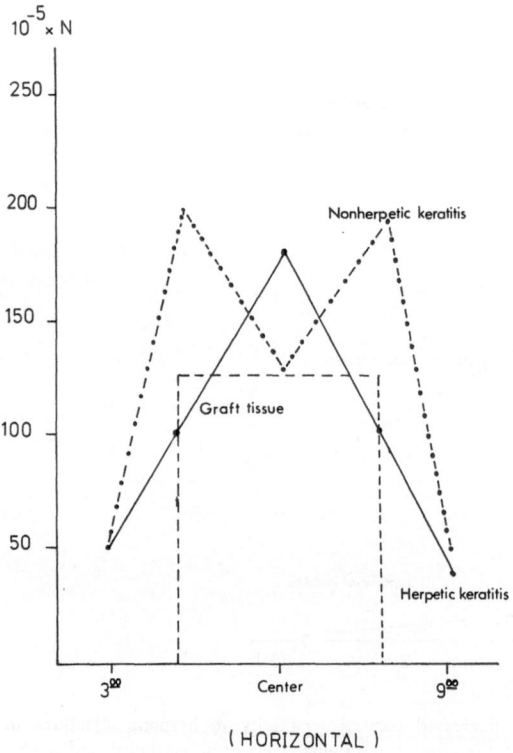

Fig. 102. Threshold after keratoplasty, for herpetic and nonherpetic corneal disease, seven years after the operation (horizontal meridian)

for a herpetic keratitis. The increase in central sensitivity is more slow and after several years the central threshold is still higher than the one in the corneal periphery. The inversion of the threshold curve persists or is only incompletely normalized. The quantitative esthesiometry with reproducible measurements is therefore a valuable examination for the differential diagnosis and the follow-up of a herpetic keratitis. In contrast to other types of keratitis the herpetic form produces not only a general lowering of corneal sensitivity, but it leads to the typical reversal of the topographic threshold curve with a marked increase of the central threshold. According to our measurements the extent of altered corneal sensitivity corresponds to the severity of the disease and the frequency of recurrences. The quantitative measurements of the threshold allow us not only to evaluate the hyposensitivity which is always present after any keratoplasty, but also other types and modes of decreased sensitivity. We are therefore in a position to measure corneal sensitivity after a keratoplasty and to note any unusual deviation in the recovery pattern. This could point to a possible recurrence of the herpetic disease, also in the graft itself.

# 23. Corneal Sensitivity
# After Trigeminal Block

The loss of corneal reflex and the subsequent neuroparalytic keratitis are of clinical importance in a patient with trigeminal neuralgia in whom the fifth nerve has been surgically severed. Trigeminal neuralgia is characterized by exquisitely painful attacks which often last only a few seconds, but may recur up to a hundred times a day. The attacks may be triggered by chewing or talking (trigger points). In secondary trigeminal neuralgias the etiology can easily be determined (e.g. tumors of the cerebellopontine angle, herpes zoster, multiple sclerosis); no etiology is found in cases of idiopathic trigeminal neuralgia (i.e. typical or genuine neuralgia). Most frequently affected are the second and third branches of the trigeminal nerve.

Medical treatment is often successful during the early stages of the disease. If this does not help, a neurosurgical procedure may be indicated: the affected trigeminal nerves may be eradicated or inactivated by the injection of alcohol, the retroganglional root may be partially severed (Spiller–Frazier) or the root of the trigeminal nerve may be cut at the cerebellopontine angle (Dandy). All of these procedures attempt to interrupt the sensory fibers in the nerve. If the procedure is successful, the typical attacks will cease. Secondary sequelae are, however, analgesia and anesthesia of the areas supplied by these trigeminal branches. There is also the danger of a neuroparalytic keratitis on the affected side. In recent years less destructive procedures have been performed, the graded thermocautery of the gasserian ganglion which is a further development of the electrocoagulation (Kirschner) and the decompression operation of the root of the trigeminal nerve (Janetta, 1971) (Freckmann, Baum, Grubel, 1982). It is an advantage of the graded thermocautery procedure that this less invasive and less radical method may be performed on patients of advanced age. This is in contrast to the older procedures.

In a pilot study we first tested the corneal sensitivity of 14 patients who had been operated on between 1967 and 1976 according to the old method of Spiller–Frazier. On an average 10.3 years had passed since the operation. The mean age of the patients was 62.9 years, the youngest patients was at the time of the follow-up examination 36 and the oldest 77 years. Ten of the 14 patients were women. In 12 patients the right trigeminal was affected and most frequently involved were the third and the second plus third branches (Table 14). All patients suffered from an idiopathic trigeminal neuralgia.

Table 14. *Vital Statistics of the 14 Patients Operated According to the Method of Frazier–Spiller (1967–1976)*

| | |
|---|---|
| Average age | 62.9 years (36–77 years) |
| Sex | 10 women= 71.4%<br>4 men   = 28.6% |
| Affected side | 12 right  = 85.7%<br>2 left   = 14.3% |

| Affected branches | | | | |
|---|---|---|---|---|
| V-1 | V-2 | V-3 | V-1.2 | V-2.3 |
| 7.1% | 14.3% | 35.7% | 7.1% | 35.7% |

| | |
|---|---|
| Loss of corneal reflex | 2 = 14.3% |
| Decreased corneal sensitivity | 4 = 28.6% |

We noticed in these patients the usual sequelae, i.e. analgesia and anesthesia or hypalgesia and hypesthesia. In two patients there was loss of corneal reflex and in four patients decreased corneal sensitivity with a slightly diminished corneal reflex. These observations could be verified by measurements with the new esthesiometer. In the two patients who lost their corneal reflex the thresholds were more than $1000 \times 10^{-5}$ N centrally and at 6:00 o'clock at the limbus. In those patients who showed a decreased corneal reflex the values were lower (central: 36.8; at 6:00 o'clock: $53 \times 10^{-5}$ N mean value), but significantly higher than in those patients who had a normal corneal reflex (central: 1.4; at 6:00 o'clock: $5.4 \times 10^{-5}$ N mean value) (see Table 15).

Table 15. *Average Corneal Sensitivity of 14 Patients Operated on According to the Procedure of Frazier–Spiller (Between 1967–1976) (in $10^{-5}$ N)*

| | Loss of reflex | | Diminished corneal sensitivity | | Normal corneal sensitivity | |
|---|---|---|---|---|---|---|
| | b | g | b | g | b | g |
| Central | >1000 | 6 | 36.8 | 7 | 1.4 | 1.5 |
| at 6:00 o'clock | >1000<br>2 patients | 3 | 53<br>4 patients | 21.3 | 5.4<br>8 patients | 4.8 |

b = Bad eye, g = Good eye.

We undertook a prospective study of corneal sensitivity in seven patients, four of whom had been untreated and three of them had a previous operation for the neuralgia. The mean age was 68.1 years, the youngest patient was 34 and the oldest patient 83. Three were women and four were men. In five patients the right trigeminal nerve was affected and V-3 or V-2+3 were again most frequently involved (Table 16).

Table 16. *Vital Statistics of Seven Patients with Trigeminal Neuralgia (1983)*

| | |
|---|---|
| Average age | 68.1 years (34–83 years) |
| Sex | 3 women = 42.9%<br>4 men  = 57.1% |
| Affected side | 5 right  = 71.4%<br>2 left  = 28.6% |

Affected branches

| V-1 | V-2 | V-3 | V-1.2 | V-2.3 |
|---|---|---|---|---|
| – | 14.3% | 57.1% | – | 28.6% |

| | |
|---|---|
| Not previously treated neuralgia | 57.1% (= 4) |
| Previously treated neuralgia | 42.9% (= 3) |

Esthesiometric examination showed that these patients did not undergo any significant change in corneal sensitivity before, five hours and four days after the graded thermocautery. There were minimal deviations (see Table 17) which, however, were within the range of normal (Draeger, Koudelka, Lubahn, 1976).

Table 17. *Mean Corneal Sensitivity in Four Patients With Untreated Trigeminal Neuralgia Before and After Controlled Thermocautery of the Gasserian Ganglion (1983) (in $10^{-5}N$)*

| | Before the operation | | Five hours after the operation | | Four days after the operation | |
|---|---|---|---|---|---|---|
| | b | g | b | g | b | g |
| Central | 1.8 | 1.0 | 2.0 | 1.0 | 2.0 | 1.0 |
| at 6:00 o'clock | 11.3 | 7.5 | 13.0 | 7.8 | 14.5 | 7.5 |

b = Bad eye, g = Good eye.

Three patients with previously treated trigeminal neuralgia were also examined before and after the controlled thermocautery. These three patients showed a diverse course and had to be evaluated individually. The youngest patient, A, (34 years old) had previously a decompression and an alcohol injection into the nerve. He showed no changes of corneal sensitivity before and after the graded thermocautery (see Table 18). Patient B (77 years old) had a thermocoagulation according to Kirschner before he underwent the graded thermocautery. He had before this operation in both eyes a slight corneal hyposensitivity with a mildly decreased corneal reflex on the right side. After the thermocautery his thresholds were in the center twice as high as before the operation; these values remained unchanged four days postoperatively. Patient C (63 years old) had previously twice a thermocoagulation of the mandibular nerve. He had before the thermocautery an average hyposensitivity. After the operation the value remained unchanged in the corneal center whereas at the 6:00 o'clock position it increased fourfold; these values also remained unchanged four days postoperatively.

Table 18. *Corneal Sensitivity in Three Patients Who Had Been Pretreated for Trigeminal Neuralgia. Values Before and After Graded Thermocautery of the Gasserian Ganglion (1983) (in $10^{-5}N$)*

|  | Before the operation | | Five hours after the operation | | Four days after the operation | |
|---|---|---|---|---|---|---|
|  | b | g | b | g | b | g |
| A. Central | 1.0 | 1.0 | 1.0 | 1.0 | 1.0 | 1.0 |
| at 6:00 o'clock | 1.0 | 1.0 | 1.0 | 1.0 | 1.0 | 1.0 |
| B. Central | 22 | 31 | 51 | 29 | 53 | 30 |
| at 6:00 o'clock | 38 | 52 | 32 | 51 | 30 | 45 |
| C. Central | 73 | 1 | 70 | 1 | 65 | 1 |
| at 6:00 o'clock | 15 | 13 | 64 | 14 | 65 | 12 |

b = Bad eye, g = Good eye.

## 23.1 Discussion

Any neurosurgical procedure on the trigeminal nerve may lead to a decreased corneal sensitivity or even to a total loss of corneal reflex and perhaps to a neuroparalytic keratitis. Up to recently it was not possible to make any definite statements as to the degree of sensitivity loss after interruption the trigeminal nerve. Boberg-Ans (1955) described for the first time measurements which were more precise than the usual method of testing corneal sensitivity with a cotton wisp. He used a modified v. Frey method. He found in 24 patients with trigeminal neuralgia normal corneal sensitivity before the operation; after the neurosurgical intervention he found "slight changes in some cases."

The new esthesiometer enables us to obtain exact data. In a pilot study we examined 14 patients who had been operated on according to the method of Spiller–Frazier; we also examined seven patients before and after a graded thermocautery. All except two patients had an idiopathic trigeminal neuralgia. The other two patients had a secondary neuralgia due to multiple sclerosis.

In four of these patients was the corneal sensitivity slightly decreased and the corneal reflex somewhat diminished; two patients had lost their corneal reflex. One of these patients gave a history of a postoperative neuroparalytic keratitis. Pothe–Usbeck reported in 1966 that such a keratitis developed in 3.8% of the patients operated according to the procedure of Spiller–Frazier. Decreased corneal sensitivity was not only observed after severing the ophthalmic branch (as would be expected), but also after interrupting the maxillary and the mandibular branches. Krayenbühl (1968) assumes that this is due to the imprecise surgical separation between the first and second branches.

Siegfried reported in 1981 that 4.4% of 135 cases developed after controlled thermocautery of the gasserian ganglion a decreased corneal sensitivity. We examined four patients before and after the thermocautery and could not find any change in sensitivity. In two of the three patients who had previously been operated on for the neuralgia, we found even before the thermocautery a decreased corneal sensitivity. This was worse after the thermocautery. We found in one of these patients loss of corneal reflex and a subsequent neuroparalytic keratitis.

It is of clinical importance that all neurosurgical interventions on the trigeminal nerve may lead to decreased corneal sensitivity and even to a loss of the corneal reflex. This applies especially to the older operative methods of partial retroganglional interruption of the root of the nerve according to Spiller and Frazier. This may lead to trophic disturbances of the cornea and even to a neuroparalytic keratitis.

The small number of our patients allows only cautious conclusions. It seems reasonable, however, to expect that in patients who had a pretreated trigeminal neuralgia, the thermocautery will in all probability lead to decreased corneal sensitivity whereas the thermocautery alone may not affect the cornea.

# 24. Conclusion

It is quite obvious that the preceding chapters are only the first step into a new exciting field of ophthalmic diagnosis. This field of exact, reproducible, quantitative corneal esthesiometry is of recent origin and we do not claim that all of its morphologic, neurophysiologic, pharmacologic and pathophysiologic aspects have been covered. The longer we have used this new examination method, the more manifold have become the various possibilities of applying it. New questions have arisen and more questions have been asked by other investigators. The testing of compounds which originally had apparently nothing to do with corneal sensitivity brought new and unexpected results. This led us into the field of human genetics and pharmacokinetic research. The numerous problems of corneal wound healing, not only in connection with keratoplasty, have not yet been exhaustively investigated. A rich harvest of clinical applications should result from these investigations. We shall continue our examinations on the possibility that corneal sensitivity may be an indicator for a beginning diabetic polyneuropathy perhaps giving us a lead as to the diabetic control. This question has not yet been completely resolved. Further investigations are necessary to evaluate the most interesting results after a surgical retinal detachment procedure. These may be of pathophysiologic and clinical importance. The same holds for the fitting of contact lenses: We may be dealing here not only with a possible predictive factor which would indicate whether the patient can tolerate a contact lens or not, but this examination method may also be of value for patients who have worn contact lenses for a long period of time. Increased thresholds could indicate a threatening complication. The use of this examination method in connection with the use of preserved corneal buttons in corneal transplant operations has opened a new field of application: In addition to the usual methods of evaluating the corneal endothelium and measuring corneal thickness, the esthesiometry may give us a further indication as to the trophic condition of the corneal transplant.

We should not forget the original domain of this examination method which Max von Frey emphasized 100 years ago: Its value for the diagnosis and follow-up examinations of herpes simplex keratitis.

Esthesiometry may help us to establish an early diagnosis and to evaluate the use of various virostatic medications. Such a quantitative evaluation method was so far not available. It was also not known that the herpes simplex infection has a varying effect on the corneal sensitivity and this may give us a hint as to the prognosis of the disease. In this connection we have to mention the surgical procedures to block the trigeminal nerve. This field is of interest to neurologists and to neurosurgeons: The considerable advances in neurosurgical technique are reflected in the much milder damage to corneal sensitivity. The surgeon can shortly after the procedure follow his results by measuring corneal sensitivity. This mean that not only the ophthalmologist (in practice and in research) will in the future use this new quantitative examination method, but it will also be most important to neurologists and neurosurgeons.

This monograph should only be a stimulus in order to motivate others to continue scientific and investigative work. This simple, quick and painless method should in the future lead us to numerous other diagnostic possibilities.

# References

Adriani, J., Zepernick, R.: Clinical effectiveness of drugs used for topical anaesthesia. JAMA *188*, 711–716 (1964).

Adriani, J., Zepernick, R., Authement, E.: The comparative potency and effectiveness of topical anaesthetics in man. Clin. Pharmacol. Therapeut. *5*, 49–62 (1964).

Armaly, M. F., Becker, B.: Intraocular pressure response to topical corticosteroids. Federation Proceedings *24*, 1274–1278 (1965).

Babel, J., Campos, R.: Sur la régénération des nerfs dans les gréffons cornéens. Ophthal. (Basel) *111*, 140–145 (1946).

Beuerman, R. W., Maurice, D. M., Tanelian, D. L.: Thermal stimulation of the cornea. In: Pain in the Trigeminal Region (Anderson, D. J., Matthews, B., eds.), pp. 413–422. Amsterdam: Elsevier. 1977.

Bigar, F., Kaufman, H. E., McCarey, B. E., Binder, P. S.: Improved corneal storage for penetrating keratoplasty in man. Am. J. Ophthal. *79*, 115–124 (1975).

Bischoff, P.: Erfahrungen mit Timolol in der Glaukomtherapie. Klin. Mbl. Augenheilk. *173*, 202–207 (1978).

Boberg-Ans, J.: Experience in clinical examination of corneal sensitivity and the nasolacrimal reflex after retrobulbar anaesthesia. Brit. J. Ophthal. *39*, 705–726 (1955).

Boberg-Ans, J.: On the corneal sensitivity. Acta ophthal. (Kbh.) *34*, 149–162 (1956).

Bonnet, R., Millodot, M.: L'esthésie cornéenne, sa mesure dans l'obscurité. Clin. Ophthal. *6*, 74–78 (1965).

Bromm, B., Treede, R. D.: Withdrawal reflex, skin resistance and reactions and pain ratings due to electrical stimuli in man. Pain *9*, 339–354 (1980).

Bryon, H. M., Weseley, A. C.: Clinical investigation of corneal contact lenses. Am. J. Ophthal. *51*, 675–694 (1961).

Brückner, R.: Schädigungen des Auges durch Medikamente. Klin. Mbl. Augenheilk. *161*, 772–786 (1973).

Büchi, J., Cordes, G., Perlia, X.: Beziehungen zwischen den physikalisch-chemischen Eigenschaften und der lokalanästhetischen Wirkung einiger Procain-Analoge. Arzneimittel-Forschung *14*, 161–169 (1964).

Buhr-Unger, H., Draeger, J., Lüders, M.: Aesthesiometrie bei Herpes corneae. Inst. Symp. Dtsch. Opthal. Ges., Freiburg, pp. 53–57. München: J. F. Bergmann. 1981.

Burgess, P. R.: Cutaneous mechanoreceptors and nociceptors. In: Handbook of Sensory Physiology, Vol. II: The Somatosensory System (Iggo, A., ed.), p. 29. Berlin-Heidelberg-New York: Springer. 1973.

Busacca, A.: Biomikroskopie und Histopathologie des Auges, Bd. 1. Zürich: Schweiz. Druck- und Verlagshaus. 1963.

Cerise, L.: De la sensibilité cornéenne. Thèse, Paris, 1908. Zit. von Schröder, E., in: v. Graefes Arch. *111*, 17–32 (1923).

Ciurlo, G.: Modificazioni della sensibilità corneale indetto degli interventi chirurgici per distacco di retina. Ann. oftal. *91*, 282–292 (1965).

Cochet, P., Bonnet, R.: L'esthésie cornéenne. Clinophthal. *4*, 3–27 (1960).

Cochet, P., Bonnet, R.: L'estésiometrie cornéenne. Réalisation et intérêt pratique. Bull. Soc. ophtal. Fr. 7, 541–550 (1961).

Conner-Moss, L.: The corneal nerves and their regeneration after surgery. Trans. Am. Ophthal. Soc. 47, 621–649 (1949).

Dandy, W. E.: Operation for cure of tic douloureux – Partial section of the root at the pons. Arch. Surg. 18, 687–734 (1929).

Daubs, J. G.: Diabetes screening with the corneal aesthesiometer. Am. J. Optom. Physiol. Optics 52, 31–34 (1975).

Dausch, D., Michelson, W., Lorenz, E. D.: Die Langzeitbehandlung des Weitwinkelglaukoms mit Timolol. Klin. Mbl. Augenheilk. 174, 127–135 (1979).

Dawson, W. W.: The thermal excitation of afferent neurones in the mammalian cornea and iris. In: Temperature. Its Measurement and Control in Science and Industry (Hardy, J. D., ed.). New York: Reinhold. 1963.

Demailly, Ph., Lehner, M. A., Duperre, J.: Un nouveau béta-bloquant dans le traitement du glaucome chronique à angle ouvert: le maléate de Timolol. J. Fr. ophtal. 1, 12, 723–731 (1978a).

Dixon, J. M.: Ocular changes due to contact lenses. Am. J. Ophthal. 58, 424–443 (1964).

Dohlmann, C. H.: Cornes and sclera. Ann. Rev. Arch. Ophthal. 71, 249–263 (1964).

Downie, A. W., Newell, D. J.: Sensory nerve conduction in patients with diabetes mellitus and controls. Neurology 11, 876–882 (1961).

Draeger, J., Richert, J.: In: Die ophthalmologischen Untersuchungsmethoden (Straub, W., Hrsg.). Stuttgart: Enke. 1970.

Draeger, J., Kudelka, A., Lubahn, E.: Zur Aesthesiometrie der Hornhaut. Klin. Mbl. Augenheilk. 169, 407–421 (1976).

Draeger, J., Martin, R.: Reinnervation der Hornhaut nach cornealen und corneoskleralen Wunden, S. 205–209. München: J. F. Bergmann. 1980.

Draeger, J.: Modern aesthesiometry: Contribution to corneal metabolism after anterior segment surgery. Trans. Ophthal. Soc. U. K. 99, 247–250 (1980).

Draeger, J., Buhr-Unger, H., Lüders, M.: Untersuchungen zur lokalanaesthetischen Wirkung der Beta-Rezeptorenblocker. Ber. dtsch. ophthal. Ges. 77, 577–581 (1980).

Draeger, J., Heid, W., Lüders, M.: Ästhesiometrie bei Kontaktlinsenträgern. Contactologia 2D, 83–93 (1980).

Draeger, J., Langenbucher, H., Lüders, M., Bannert, Ch.: Zur Wirkung von Oberflächenanaesthetika am Auge. Klin. Mbl. Augenheilk. 177, 780–788 (1980).

Draeger, J., Buhr-Unger, H., Winter, R.: Die Wirkung von Beta-Rezeptoren-Blockern auf die Hornhautsensibilität, pp. 195–199. München: J. F. Bergmann. 1982.

Draeger, J., Schneider, B., Winter, R.: Die lokalanästhetische Wirkung von Metipranolol im Vergleich zu Timolol. Klin. Mbl. Augenheilk. 182, 210–213 (1983).

Draeger, J., Winter, R.: Die lokalanästhetische Wirkung von Metipranolol im Vergleich zu Timolol bei augengesunden Patienten. In: Metipranolol, pp. 76–84. Wien-New York: Springer. 1983.

Draeger, J., Winter, R.: Corneal sensitivity and intraocularpressure. In: Glaucoma Update, pp. 63–70. Berlin-Heidelberg-New York: Springer. 1983.

Duke-Elder, S.: System of ophthalmology, Vol. II, IV and VI. London: Kimpton. 1968.

Edinger, H., Schloot, W., Goedde, H. W.: Zum Polymorphismus der sauren Erythrozytenphosphatase; Untersuchung zur formalen Genetik und zur Populationsgenetik in Thailand. Z. Morph. Anthrop. 66, 217–231 (1975).

Ehlers, N.: The precorneal film. Acta ophthal. (Kbh.) Suppl. 81, 5–136 (1965).

Emmerich, R., Carter, G. Z., Berens, C.: An experimental clinical evaluation of dorsacaine hydrochloride (Benoxinate Novesine). Am. J. Ophthal. 40, 841–848 (1955).

Escapini, M.: Degeneration and regeneration of nerves in corneal transplantation. Arch. Ophthal. *39*, 135–161 (1948).

Forsius, H.: Sensitivity of the cornea in arcus senilis. Acta ophthal. (Kbh.) *36*, 43–49 (1958).

Franceschetti, A.: Examen histologique d'une grèffe cornéenne transparente: Le comportement des nerfs. Ann. ocul. *180*, 142–145 (1947).

Freckmann, N., Baum, H., Grubel, G.: Die Behandlung der sogenannten idiopathischen Trigeminusneuralgie heute. HÄB *7*, 234–236 (1982).

von Frey, M.: Beiträge zur Physiologie des Schmerzes. In: Berichte über die Verhandlungen der Königlich sächsischen Gesellschaft der Wissenschaften zu Leipzig, Mathematische Classe, pp. 185–196. Leipzig: Hirzel. 1894.

von Frey, M., Strughold, H.: Weitere Untersuchungen über das Verhalten von Hornhaut und Bindehaut des menschlichen Auges gegen Berührungsreize. Ztschr. f. Biol. *84*, 321–334 (1926).

Goecke, G, Schwabe, G.: Vorschläge einer Stadieneinteilung der Gestose. Zbl. Gynäk. *87*, 1439–1443 (1965).

Goldschneider, A., Brückner, A.: Zur Physiologie des Schmerzes. Die Sensibilität der Hornhaut des Auges. Berl. Klin. Wschr. *52*, 1225–1226 (1919).

Gotz, R.: Zwei neue Instrumente für die Untersuchung der Hornhautsensibilität. Klin. Mbl. Augenheilk. *161*, 469–474 (1972).

Grüter, W.: Die Ätiologie der Keratitis disciformis. Ber. dtsch. ophthal. Ges. *48*, 209–211 (1930).

Günther, G.: Spätergebnisse der Keratoplastik an 100 erfolgreichen Transplantationen. Ber. dtsch. ophthal. Ges. *64*, 159–164 (1961).

Hamano, H.: Topical and systemic influences of wearing contact lenses. Contacto *4*, 41–48 (1960).

Hardenberger, R., Hanna, C., Boyd, C.: Effects of drug vehicles on ocular contact time. Arch. Ophthal. *93*, 42–45 (1975).

Hayes, A. D., Barber, P.: Ultrastructure of the corneal nerves in the rat. Cell Tissue Res. *172*, 133–144 (1976).

Hogan, M.: Histology of the Human Eye. An Atlas and Textbook. Philadelphia-London-Toronto: Saunders. 1971.

Janetta, P. J.: Vascular decompression in trigeminal neuralgia. In: The Cranial Nerves (Samii, M., Janetta, P. J., eds.), pp. 331–340. Berlin-Heidelberg-New York: Springer. 1981.

Kalfa, S. F., Paramonov, A. F.: Veränderungen der Empfindlichkeit in der Zone des ersten und des zweiten Astes des Nervus trigeminus bei Glaukom. Vest. oftal. (Mosk.) *34*, 33–37 (1955).

Kemmetmüller, H.: Corneal sensitivity and contact lens fitting. F. ophthal. Jap. *20*, Suppl. 7–12 (1969).

Kenshalo, D. R., et al.: Comparison of thermal sensitivity of the forehead, lip, conjunctiva and cornea. J. Appl. Physiol. *15*, 987–991 (1960).

Kirschner, M.: Elektrokoagulation des Ganglion Gasseri. Zbl. Chir. *47*, 2841–2842 (1932).

Klingmüller, O.: Untersuchungen über die Zusammensetzung und Wirkung von wäßrigen Augenarzneien. Dissertation, Hamburg, 1957.

Kornblueth, W., Maumenee, E., Crowell, J. E.: Regeneration of nerves in experimental corneal grafts in rabbits. Am. J. Ophthal. *32*, 651–658 (1949).

Krayenbühl, H.: Die ichiopathische Trigeminusneuralgie. Doc. Geigy, acta clinica *9*, 12–13, 24, 36 (1968).

Krieglstein, G. K., Sold-Darseff, J., Leydhecker, W.: The intraocular pressure response of glaucomatous eyes to topically applied Bupranolol. A pilot study. Albrecht von Graefe's Arch. ophthal. *202*, 81–86 (1977).

Krieglstein, G. K.: Die Wirkung von Timolol-Augentropfen auf den Augeninnendruck. Klin. Mbl. Augenheilk. *172*, 677–685 (1978).

Krückmann, E.: v. Graefes Arch. Ophthal. *41*, Abt. 4, 21 (1895). [Ref.: Severin, M.: Klin. Mbl. Augenheilk. *146*, 683–695 (1965).]

Kuschinsky, G., Lüllmann, H.: Kurzes Lehrbuch der Pharmakologie. Stuttgart: G. Thieme. 1976.

Lands, A. M., Arnold, J. P., Auliff, M. C.: Differentiation of receptor systems activated by sympathomimetic amines. Nature *214*, 597–598 (1967).

Larke, J. R., Hirji, N. K.: Some clinically observed phenomena in extended contact lens wear. Brit. J. Ophthal. *63*, 475–477 (1979).

Larson, W. L.: Electro-mechanical corneal aesthesiometer. Brit. J. Ophthal. *54*, 342–347 (1970).

Lele, P. P., Weddell, G.: The relationship between neurohistology and corneal sensitivity. Brain *79*, 119–154 (1956).

Lele, P. P., Weddell, G.: Sensory nerves of the cornea and cutaneous sensibility. Exper. Neurol. *1*, 334–359 (1959).

Lemp, M. A., Holly, F. J.: Ophthalmic polymers as ocular wetting agents. Ann. Ophthal. *4*, 15–20 (1972).

Linn, J. G., Vey, E. K.: Topic anaesthesia in ophthalmology. Am. J. Ophthal. *40*, 697–704 (1955).

Luchik, V. J.: Results of an investigation into sensitiveness of the cornea in normal and glaucomatous eyes by using Radziphorsky's method. Vestn. oftal. *79*, 51–55 (1966).

Lyne, A. J.: Corneal sensation in scleritis and episcleritis. Brit. J. Ophthal. *61*, 650–654 (1977).

McCarey, B. E.: Improved corneal storage. Invest. Ophthal. *13*, 165–173 (1974).

Marinosci, A.: Sulla sensibilità della cornea allo stato normale a patologico. Lett. oftalm. *7*, 407–423 (1930).

Mark, D., Maurice, D. M.: Sensory recording from the isolated cornea. Invest. Ophthal. *16*, 541–545 (1977).

Marx, E.: Die Empfindlichkeit der menschlichen Hornhaut. Leipzig: Hirzel. 1925.

Maumenee, A. E., Kornblueth, W.: Symposion: Corneal transplantation IV. Physiopathology (1949).

Maurice, D. M.: The permeability of Sodium ions of the living rabbits cornea. J. Physiol. *122*, 367–387 (1951).

Maurice, D. M.: The structure and transparency of the cornea. J. Physiol. *136*, 263–286 (1957).

Mensher, J. H.: Corneal nerves. Survey of Ophthal. *19*, 1–18 (1974).

Millodot, M., Larson, W.: Effect of bending of the nylon thread of the Cochet-Bonnet corneal aesthesiometer upon the recorded pressure. Contact Lens *1*, 5–7 (1967).

Millodot, M.: Corneal sensitivity and contact lenses. The Optician *162*, 23–24 (1971).

Millodot, M.: Diurnal variation of the cornea sensivitity. Brit. J. Ophthal. *56*, 844–847 (1972).

Millodot, M.: Objective measurement of corneal sensitivity. Acta Ophthal. (Kbh.) *51*, 325–334 (1973).

Millodot, M.: Effect of soft lenses on corneal sensitivity. Acta Ophthal. (Kbh.) *52*, 603–608 (1974).

Millodot, M.: Effect of the length of wear of contact lenses on corneal sensitivity. Acta Ophthal. (Kbh.) *54*, 721–730 (1976).

Millodot, M.: The influence of pregnancy of the sensitivity of the cornea. Brit. J. Ophthal. *61*, 646–649 (1977).

Millodot, M.: Does the long term wear of contact lenses produce a loss of corneal sensitivity. Experientia *33*, 1475–1476 (1977).

Morales-Aguilera, A., Williams, E. M.: The effect on cardiac muscle of betareceptor antagonists in relation to their activity as local anaesthetics. Brit. J. Pharmacol. *24*, 332–338 (1965).

Morinaga, T.: Acta Soc. Ophthal. Jap. *35*, 511, 544 (1931). [Zit. von Heydenreich, J., in: Der Augenarzt, Bd. II. Stuttgart: G. Thieme. 1931.]

Moses, R. A., Cotlier, E.: The cornea. In: Adler's Physiology of the eye. St. Louis: Mosby. 1970.

Müller, H. K., Söllner, F., Vucicevic, Z.: Spätergebnisse bei der Keratoplastik. Ber. dtsch. ophthal. Ges. *64*, 142–159 (1961).

Mummenthaler, M.: Neurologie. Stuttgart: G. Thieme. 1982.

Nafe, J., Wagoner, K.: Sensitivity of cornea to heat and pain derived from high temperatures. Am. J. Psychol. *49*, 631–635 (1937).

Nielsen, N. V.: Corneal sensitivity and vibratory perception in diabetes mellitus. Acta ophthal. *56*, 406–411 (1978).

Nielsen, N. V.: Timolol. Hypotensive effect, used alone and in combination for treatment of increased ocular pressure. Acta ophthal. *56*, 504–511 (1978).

Norn, M. S.: Dendritic (herpetic) keratitis. IV. Follow-up examination of corneal sensitivity. Acta ophthal. *48*, 383–395 (1970).

Norn, M. S.: Conjunctival sensitivity in normal eyes. Acta ophthal. *51*, 325–334 (1973).

Ophthalmica: Eine Monographie der Arbeitsgemeinschaft für Pharmazeutische Verfahrenstechnik e. V., Mainz. Stuttgart: Wissenschaftliche Verlagsgesellschaft. 1975.

Pandolfi, M., Öhrström, A.: Treatment of ocular hypertension with oral beta-adrenergic blocking agents. Acta ophthal. *52*, 464–467 (1974).

Pannarale, M. R., Pannarale, C.: Rilievi sulla sensibilità corneale negli operati di distacco retinico. Bull. Oculist. *44*, 929–943 (1965).

Perl, E. R.: Is pain a specific sensation? J. Psychiatr. Res. *8*, 273–287 (1971).

Pflimlin, R.: Zur klinischen Unterscheidung verschiedener Formen des Herpes corneae. Dtsch. Ophthal. Ges., p. 212 (1930).

Phillips, C., Howitt, G., Rowlands, D. J.: Propranolol as ocular hypotensive agent. Brit. J. Ophthal. *51*, 222–226 (1967).

Pöntinen, P. J., Miettinen, P.: Neuroleptanalgesia in cataract surgery, Part I. Acta ophthal., Suppl. 80 (1964).

Pöntinen, P. J., Miettinen, P., Reinikainen, M.: Neuroleptangalgesia in cataract surgery, Part II. Acta ophthal., Suppl. 80 (1966).

Pothe, H., Usbeck, W.: Zur Diagnostik und Therapie der Trigeminusneuralgie unter besonderer Berücksichtigung der Operation nach Spiller–Frazier. Dtsch. med. Wschr. *52*, 2330–2361 (1966).

Radzichovskij, B. L.: Magnety alegesimeter. (Magnetisches Algesimeter). Vest. oftal. (Mosk.) *2*, 81–82 (1971).

Reiser, K. A.: Durch welche histologischen Veränderungen ist die Sensibilitätsstörung der Cornea beim Herpes zu erklären? Klin. Mbl. Augenheilk. *104*, 257–263 (1940).

Rexed, B., Rexed, U.: Degeneration and regeneration of corneal nerves. Brit. J. Ophthal. *35*, 38–49 (1951).

Rexed, U.: Nerve regeneration in corneal grafts in the rabbit. Brit. J. Ophthal. *35*, 89–97 (1950).

Rintelen, F.: Augenheilkunde. Basel-New York: Karger. 1969.

Ritchie, J. M., Cohen, P. J.: Local anaesthetics. In: Basis of Therapeutics (Goodman, L. S., Gilman, A., eds.). New York: Macmillan. 1975.

Rogell, G. D.: Internal ophthalmoplegia after argon laserpanretinal photocoagulation. Arch. Ophthal. *97*, 904–905 (1979).

Rohen, J. W.: Das Auge und seine Hilfsorgane. In: Handbuch der mikroskopischen Anatomie des Menschen, Bd. 3, Tl. 4. Berlin-Göttingen-Heidelberg-New York: Springer. 1964.

Rohen, J. W.: Die Hornhaut. Der Präcornealfilm. In: Augenheilkunde in Klinik und Praxis, Bd. 1 (François, J., Hollwich, F., eds.). Stuttgart: G. Thieme. 1977.

Ruben, M., Colebrook, E.: Keratoplasty sensitivity. Brit. J. Ophthal. 63, 265–267 (1979).

Schirmer, K. E., Mellor, S. T.: Corneal sensitivity after cataract extraction. A.M.A. Arch. Ophthal. 65, 433–437 (1961).

Schirmer, K. E.: Assessment of corneal sensitivity. Brit. J. Ophthal. 47, 488–492 (1963).

Schloot, W., Goedde, H. W.: Biochemische Genetik des Menschen. In: Handbuch der Allgemeinen Pathologie Erbgefüge (Vogel, F., ed.). Berlin-Heidelberg-New York: Springer. 1974.

Schloot, W., Goedde, H. W.: Psychopharmakogenetik. Med. Klin. 71, 481–495 (1976).

Schloot, W.: Praktische Aspekte der Pharmakogenetik. Monatskurs f. d. ärztl. Fortbildung 2, 78–81 (1978).

Schröder, E.: Prüfung der Hornhautempfindlichkeit nach operativen Eingriffen. v. Graefes Arch. Ophthal. 111, 17–32 (1923).

Schwartz, D. E.: Corneal sensitivity in diabetics. Arch. Ophthal. 91, 174–178 (1974).

Sedan, J.: Bericht über zwei Fälle von Unterempfindlichkeit der Hornhaut, festgestellte 3 Jahre nach retrobulbärer Injektion von Acetylcholin. Bull. Soc. ophtal. France 340–343 (1957).

Severin, M.: Die Hornhautsensibilität bei herpetischer Keratitis. Klin. Mbl. Augenheilk. 146, 683–695 (1965).

Siegfried, J.: Percutaneous controlled thermocoagulation of Gasserian ganglion in trigeminal neuralgie. In: The Cranial Nerves (Samii, M., Janetta, P. J., eds.), pp. 322–330. Berlin-Heidelberg-New York: Springer. 1981.

Simkova, M.: Über die Therapie der herpetischen Erkrankungen des Auges. Therapie mit Gynergen und „Dihydroergotamin Sandoz". Ophthal. (Basel) 119, 381–396 (1950).

Snow, J. C., Sensel, S.: A review of cataract extraction under local and general anaesthesia. Anaesthesia and analgesia, Current Researches 45, 742–747 (1966).

Soehring, K., Klingmüller, O., Neuwald, F.: Pharmakologische Untersuchungen über den Einfluß der Zusammensetzung des Vehikels auf die Wirkung wäßriger Lösungen von Augenarzneien. Arzneimittel-Forschung 9, 297–305 (1959).

Spiller, W. G., Frazier, C. H.: The division of the trigeminus for the relief of the tic douloureux. Univ. Pum. Med. Bull. 14, 341–351 (1901).

Stichartz, G.: Molecular mechanisms of nerve block by local anaesthetics. Anaesthesiology 45, 421–441 (1976).

Stiegler, G.: Bupranolol-Augentropfen in der Glaukom-Dauer-Therapie. Klin. Mbl. Augenheilk. 174, 267–275 (1979).

Strughold, H.: Mechanical threshold of cornea-reflex of the usual laboratory animals. Am. J. Physiol. 94, 235–240 (1930).

Sugita, S.: Versuche mit dem „Luftstrahlaesthesiometer". Persönliche Mitteilung, 1977.

Thoma, K.: Biopharmazie der Augenarzneimittel. Pharm. Ztg. 41, 1809–1813 (1977).

Trenberth, S. M., Mishima, S.: The effect of Ouabein on the rabbit corneal endothelium. Invest. ophthal. 7, 44–52 (1968).

Trimarchi, F.: La sensibilità corneale alle variazioni termiche. Annali di ott. e clin. oculistica 99, 592–598 (1967).

Troll, W.: Investigation into the sensitivity of the human eye to hypo and hypertonic solutions as well as solutions with unphysiological hydrogen ion concentrations. Pharm. Wbl. (Amsterdam) 93, 108–148 (1958).

Umbdenstock, R.: Les Eroubles de la sensibilité cornéenne dans la kératide disciform. Bull. Soc. opht. France 1949, 964–965.

Vale, J., Gibbs, A. C. C., Phillips, C. I.: Topical propranolol and ocular tension in the human eye. Brit. J. Ophthal. *56*, 770–775 (1972).

Velhagen, K.: Senile Hornhautveränderungen. In: Der Augenarzt, Bd. III, pp. 919–920. Leipzig: VEB G. Thieme. 1975.

Waldeyer, A.: Anatomie des Menschen, Bd. 2. Berlin-New York: De Gruyter. 1975.

Waltman, S. R.: The cornea. In: Adler's Physiology of the Eye (Moses, R. A., ed.), p. 38. St. Louis-Toronto-London: Mosby. 1981.

Zander, E., Weddell, G.: Observation on the innervation of the cornea. J. Anat. Lond. *85*, 68–99 (1951).

Zander, E., Weddell, G.: Reaction of corneal nerve fibers to injury. Brit. J. Ophthal. *35*, 61–88 (1955).

Zimmerman, T. J., Kaufman, H. E.: Timolol, a beta-adrenergic blocking agent for the treatment of glaucoma. Arch. Ophthal. *95*, 601–607 (1977).

Zistl, A., Draeger, J., Drescher, K., Timm, J., Schloot, W.: Altersabhängige geschlechtsspezifische Unterschiede der Corneasensibilität. 16. Tg., Ges. Anthropol. Humangen., p. 26, Heidelberg, 29. September 1979.

Zistl, A., Draeger, J., Drescher, K., Timm, J., Schloot, W.: Aesthesiometrische Untersuchungen zum Einfluß endogener und exogener Faktoren auf die Corneasensibilität. Antrop. Anz. *40*, 101–110 (1982).

Zorab, E. C.: Corneal sensitivity after grafting. Proc. roy. Soc. Med. *64*, 117–118 (1971).

# Subject Index

# Metipranolol

Pharmacology of Beta-blocking Agents and Use
of Metipranolol in Ophthalmology
Contributions to the First Metipranolol Symposium, Berlin 1983

Edited by H.-J. Merté

1984. 73 figures (one in color). Approx. 180 pages.
ISBN 3-211-81824-3.

When a compound and its various effects are discovered there is
still a long way ahead until it is available as a finished product.
Before it reaches the physicist, the substance is examined in a
research sequence by chemists, pharmacologists, and pharmacists
— just to mention a few of the most important stages. As a result of
such extensive research and development work a new antiglauco-
matous product containing the beta-blocking compound metipranolol was presented in 1982. A series of investigators at many different
centers participated in this work and, at the invitation of Messrs. Dr.
Gerhard Mann, the manufacturers, came together for discussions at
a symposium held in Berlin in January 1983, reporting on the experiences they had made with the new substance. As the contributions
were of great interest and practical importance, it was decided to
make them generally available as a book. This book has met with
great interest and has been very readily accepted, as it fills a gap in
the literature on beta-blocking agents.

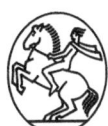

Springer-Verlag Wien New York